Drug Repurposing Against SARS-CoV-2

Edited by

Tabish Qidwai
Faculty of Biotechnology
Shri Ramswaroop Memorial University
Lucknow-Deva Road U.P.
India

Drug Repurposing Against SARS-CoV-2

Editor: Tabish Qidwai

ISBN (Online): 978-981-5123-19-7

ISBN (Print): 978-981-5123-20-3

ISBN (Paperback): 978-981-5123-21-0

Published by Bentham Science Publishers Pte. Ltd. Singapore. All Rights Reserved.

First published in 2023.

need for a court order if at any point you breach any terms of this License Agreement. In no event will any delay or failure by Bentham Science Publishers in enforcing your compliance with this License Agreement constitute a waiver of any of its rights.

3. You acknowledge that you have read this License Agreement, and agree to be bound by its terms and conditions. To the extent that any other terms and conditions presented on any website of Bentham Science Publishers conflict with, or are inconsistent with, the terms and conditions set out in this License Agreement, you acknowledge that the terms and conditions set out in this License Agreement shall prevail.

Bentham Science Publishers Pte. Ltd.
80 Robinson Road #02-00
Singapore 068898
Singapore
Email: subscriptions@benthamscience.net

BENTHAM
SCIENCE

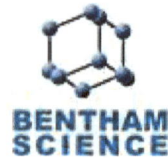

CONTENTS

FOREWORD

Drug repurposing is a process of identifying new uses of approved or investigated drugs. In the current scenario of deadly contagious coronavirus disease 2019 (COVID-19), where no specific treatment options are available, drug repurposing is considered a very effective drug discovery strategy and could be considered the new avenue for the treatment of COVID-19. The book entitled **"Drug Repurposing against SARS-CoV2"** offers comprehensive and systematic coverage of repurposed and adjuvant drugs highlighting their therapeutic status in COVID-19 patients while assessing the challenges and ethical issues related to repurposing drugs.

The pathophysiology of SARS-CoV2 replication in COVID-19 and their modulation by repurposing drugs is explained in simple and lucid language and also through enriched illustrations. The wealth of information assembled by the authors will be useful to both Pharmacologists and Clinicians.

Uma Bhandari
Department of Pharmacology
School of Pharmaceutical Education and Research (SPER)
Jamia Hamdard
India

PREFACE

There are seven chapters in this book entitled " Drug Repurposing against SARS-CoV2." The book focuses on current trends in drug repurposing against SARS-CoV2.

The goal of this book is to give readers an overview of drug repurposing in life-threating diseases, drug repurposing in COVID-19, as well as various techniques involved in drug repurposing. The book aims to target students, research scholars, and physicians interested in the topic. The book's structure is well-organized and updated.

Chapter 1 by Ruchi Chawla discusses repurposing drugs: a new paradigm and hopes for life-threatening diseases.

Anand *et al.*, in Chapter 2, outline the repurposed and adjuvant drugs in COVID-19 patients, as well as challenges and ethical issues related to drug repurposing. Chapter 3 by Neelam *et al.* presents the repurposed drugs against SARS-CoV-2 replication in COVID-19. In Chapter 4, Awesh Yadav *et al.*, describe the targeting of viral entry pathways through repurposed drugs in SARS-CoV-2 infection.

Repurposed drugs or potential pharmacological agents targeting cytokine release, and induction of coagulation in COVID-19 are discussed in Chapter 5 by Arpita Singh *et al*. In Chapter 6, Qidwai *et al.*, discuss the High-throughput screening (HTS) method for screening of known drugs. The last chapter by Khan *et al.*, discusses drug repurposing for COVID-19 using computational methods.

I believe this book will be of tremendous interest to students, doctors, researchers, and even patients and their families. Finally, I would like to express my gratitude to all of the contributors to this book, as well as the Bentham Publishing Editorial Board for providing us with this invaluable opportunity.

Tabish Qidwai
Faculty of Biotechnology, IBST
Shri Ramswaroop Memorial University
Lucknow-Deva Road
Barabanki, 225003
U.P. India

List of Contributors

Ajay Kumar Verma	Department of Respiratory Medicine, King George's Medical University, Lucknow, Uttar Pradesh, India
Anand Kumar Maurya	Department of Microbiology, All India Insititue of Medical Sciences, Bhopal, Madhya Pradesh, India
Amit Kumar Palai	Department of Pharmaceutics, National Institute of Pharmaceutical Education and Research (NIPER) Raebareli, Lucknow, Uttar Pradesh, India
Anuj Kumar Pandey	Department of Respiratory Medicine, King George's Medical University, Lucknow, Uttar Pradesh, India
Anjali Bhosale	Department of Pharmaceutics, National Institute of Pharmaceutical Education and Research (NIPER) Raebareli, Lucknow, Uttar Pradesh, India
Arpita Singh	Department of Pharmacology, Dr. Ram Manohar Lohia Institute of Medical Sciences, Lucknow, Uttar Pradesh, India
Awesh K. Yadav	Department of Pharmaceutics, National Institute of Pharmaceutical Education and Research (NIPER) Raebareli, Lucknow, Uttar Pradesh, India
Farhan Mazahir	Department of Pharmaceutics, National Institute of Pharmaceutical Education and Research (NIPER) Raebareli, Lucknow, Uttar Pradesh, India
Feroz Khan	CSIR-CIMAP, Lucknow-226015, UP, India
Jyoti Bajpai	Department of Respiratory Medicine, King George's Medical University, Lucknow, Uttar Pradesh, India
Kavita Verma	Department of Biochemistry, Dr. Rammanohar Lohia Avadh University, Ayodhya-224001, India
Krishan Kumar	Department of Pharmaceutical Engineering & Technology, Indian Institute of Technology, Varanasi-221005, India
Manisha Mulchandani	Department of Pharmaceutics, National Institute of Pharmaceutical Education and Research (NIPER) Raebareli, Lucknow, Uttar Pradesh, India
Malti Dadheech	Department of Microbiology, All India Institute of Medical Sciences, Bhopal, India
Mohini Mishra	Department of Pharmaceutical Engineering & Technology, Indian Institute of Technology, Varanasi-221005, India
Neha Kapoor	Department of Chemistry, Hindu College, University of Delhi-110007, Delhi, India
Neelam Yadav	Department of Biochemistry, Dr. Rammanohar Lohia Avadh University, Ayodhya-224001, India
Om Prakash	CSIR-CIMAP, Lucknow-226015, UP, India
Ruchi Chawla	Department of Pharmaceutical Engineering & Technology, Indian Institute of Technology, Varanasi-221005, India
Sarika Singh	Neurosciences an Ageing Biology and Toxicology and Experimental Medicine Division, CSIR-Central Drug Research Institute, Lucknow-226031, India

Tabish Qidwai   Faculty of Biotechnology, Shriramswaroop Memorial University, Lucknow, UP, India

Tejal Shreeya   Institute of Biophysics, Biological Research Centre, Szeged, Hungary, Europe

Varsha Rani   Department of Pharmaceutical Engineering & Technology, Indian Institute of Technology, Varanasi-221005, India

Yoganchal Mishra   Department of Biochemistry, Dr. Rammanohar Lohia Avadh University, Ayodhya-224001, India

CHAPTER 1

Repurposing Drugs: A New Paradigm and Hopes for Life-threatening Diseases

Ruchi Chawla[1,*], **Varsha Rani**[1], **Krishan Kumar**[1] and **Mohini Mishra**[1]

[1] *Department of Pharmaceutical Engineering & Technology, Indian Institute of Technology, Varanasi-221005, India*

Abstract: The process of repurposing drugs is an alternative to the conventional drug discovery process. It is a cost-effective and time-efficient process with high returns and low risk that utilizes mechanistic information of the existing drugs to investigate their novel applications against other disease conditions. The most significant benefit of drug repositioning is that it brings new life against novel/ orphan/ resistant diseases and pandemic outbreaks like COVID-19. As a result, widespread use of the drug repurposing strategy will not only aid in the more efficient fight against pandemics but will also combat life-threatening diseases. Therefore, repurposing drugs can provide a quick response to these unpredictable situations. In this chapter, we have tried to focus on various drug-repurposing strategies along with therapeutics for repurposing drugs against life-threatening diseases wherein little or no treatment is readily available.

Keywords: Drug-repurposing, Life-threatening diseases, New drug development, Phenotype screening.

INTRODUCTION

Drug repositioning is an alternative approach in drug development that opens new avenues for diseases wherein there is lack of appropriate treatment approaches. Drug repositioning (also known as drug repurposing, drug reprofiling, or drug re-tasking) is the process of identifying new modes of action, new indications, as well as new targets for already approved drugs or investigational drugs which have not been mentioned in any of the existing medical indications [1]. The availability of pre-clinical and clinical data allows for effective repurposing and the possibility of failure is relatively low in comparison to that of a new drug. As a result, the repurposed medicinal products require less time for clinical trials and regulatory approval [2]. The process of repurposing provides an abridged route to

---

* **Corresponding author Ruchi Chawla:** Department of Pharmaceutical Engineering & Technology, Indian Institute of Technology, BHU, Varanasi-221001, India; E-mails: ruchibits@gmail.com; rchawla.phe@iitbhu.ac.in

Tabish Qidwai (Ed.)

the conventional drug discovery process. It is a cost-effective and time-efficient process with high returns and low risk that utilizes mechanistic information of the existing drugs to investigate their novel application against other diseases and pathological conditions [3]. The most significant benefit of drug repositioning is that it brings new life against novel, orphan, resistant diseases and pandemic outbreaks like COVID-19. As a result, widespread use of the drug repurposing strategy will not only aid in the more efficient fight against pandemics but will also combat life-threatening diseases [4].

Life-threatening diseases are chronic, mainly debilitating diseases that significantly reduce a person's life expectancy. Major life-threatening diseases include cancer, diabetes, neurological conditions, coronary cardiovascular conditions and HIV/Aids [5], which are significantly impacting the global health economy. These life-threatening diseases can be prevented and treated, however, at times there is lack of response from the existing therapy. There might be a need for an alternative therapeutic regimen wherein, repurposing drugs can provide a potential backup for the same [4]. Sometimes, there are unexpected pandemics when life-threatening conditions emerge and no treatment is available, and under such circumstances, repurposition of drug products could be helpful. The majority of drugs currently repositioned in the market are a result of serendipity. The well-known cardiovascular benefits of aspirin are among one of the most appropriately proven examples of repurposing. The results of clinical trial shifted the use of sildenafil from coronary artery disease to erectile dysfunction. Bupropion was initially developed as an antidepressant before its application in cessation of smoking. Botox (on botulinum toxin A) which was first used to treat eye muscle disorders, is currently having a widespread application in cosmetic and beauty industry. Minoxidil was used to treat high blood pressure prior to the discovery of its effect on hair growth. Thalidomide and its extracts have been repurposed to treat leprosy, multiple myeloma, myelodysplastic syndrome, mantle cell lymphoma, and metastatic prostate cancer [6, 7].

New drug development is a challenging process requiring enormous investment of money and time, with unpredictable return on investment [1]. *De novo* drug development takes around 10 to 15 years, which includes basic discovery, design of medicines, *in vitro* and *in vivo* studies (including safety and efficacy), clinical studies and ultimately market registration of drugs. In contrast, repurposing medication for life-threatening diseases takes only 5-11 years, as many intermediary steps are bypassed if the therapeutic potential of the drug for the disease is confirmed as shown in Fig. (**1**) [8, 9]. This approach provides several benefits over conventional drug development with lower costs in a shorter timeframe with fewer risks, as the effectiveness and safety of the original medication have already been established and approved by regulatory agencies

[4]. In this chapter, we will highlight various drug-repurposing strategies along with therapeutics for repurposing drugs against life-threatening diseases where little or no treatment is available.

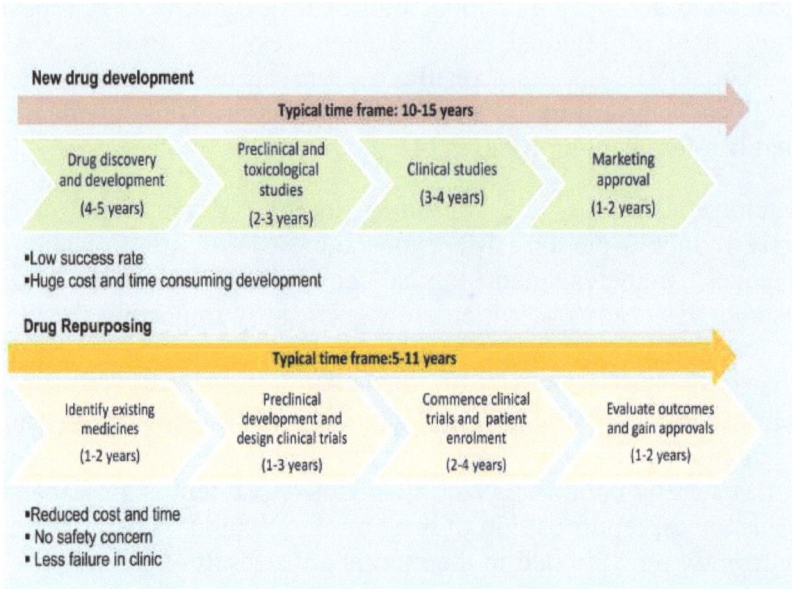

Fig. (1). The approximate time and major steps in the process of *de novo* drug development and repurposing of drugs.

Drug Repurposing Strategies

The primary objective of the drug discovery and development is to establish the therapeutic effectiveness with a very low toxicity-to-benefit ratio. As a result, strategies that use drug candidates with known therapeutic profiles (for drug repurposing) can significantly contribute to the drug development process, thereby reducing development time and costs. Drug candidates with known safety profiles can typically be selected from (a) approved FDA drugs, (b) drugs being studied for a different application, or (c) drugs abandoned or unsuccessful in clinical trials (phase II or III). The success of drug repositioning depends on maximizing therapeutic effectiveness for new targets while reducing off-target effects [10].

Repositioning of drugs is not a new concept, what is new is the ability to do it in a systematic and rational manner rather than relying on serendipity. As the prominence of drug repositioning is gaining practical applications, a number of companies are shifting their focus on developing strategies to make it a systematic exercise. Before moving the applicant drug further down the development pipeline, a drug repurposing strategy usually consists of three steps; (1) Identifying a drug applicant molecule for a new indication (hypothesis generation for new target), (2) Investigation of drug or disease-related mechanisms or signalling pathways, (3) Evaluation of Phase II and III clinical trials for efficacy (assuming that the phase I studies conducted during the original indication provides sufficient safety data). The selection of the appropriate drug for a given indication is the most important of all the mentioned steps, and it is here that modern approaches to hypothesis generation may be most useful [2]. Since the initial success of drug repurposing, several new methods for determining and validating ideas of repurposing drug targets have been developed and proposed. These repurposing approaches are frequently classified as experimental, clinical, or computational as shown in Fig. (2) [2].

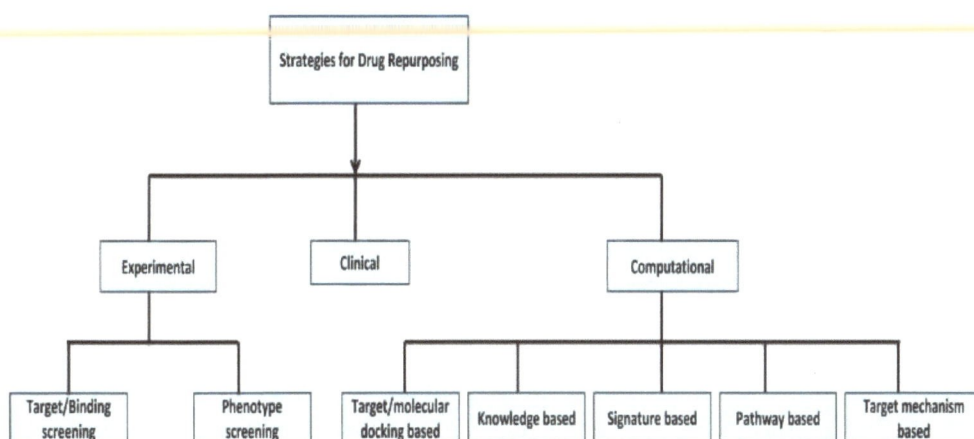

Fig. (2). Various drug-repurposing approaches: experimental, clinical and computational approaches.

Experimental Approaches

Experimental drug screening approaches include target associated screening (binding assay for identification of target candidates) and phenotype-based screening as shown in Fig. (3) [11]. In drug repurposing, during experimental screening, multiple molecules are tested through pharmacological assays against certain or more targets or phenotypes. This broad approach is based on the concept that the more is the number of compounds tested, the more is the confidence in the repositioning of the drug candidates, of which the promising ones can be passed for in depth experimental testing. Both drug development and drug repurposing utilize experimental screening approaches to discover hits, but there are substantial variations in their application and results. Although the percentage of positive hits remains low (out of the overall screened compounds), comparatively low cost is involved thus making this a successful repurposing strategy [11]. Drug discovery process usually investigates *de novo* hits that are generated *via* high throughput screening, which considers highly specialized screens and multi-million-compound libraries. As against this, during repurposing in-depth screening of smaller compounds libraries is done, which are either approved compounds or failed compounds having some information on their safety and mechanism of action (MoA). There are approximately 500-2000 compounds available in approved compound libraries, with an equal number of unapproved compounds. Some may include annotations as well as information on safety and MoA. Compound libraries are managed by drug discovery laboratories and academics which open up possibilities for identifying the hits of drug candidates for a clinical development programme [12].

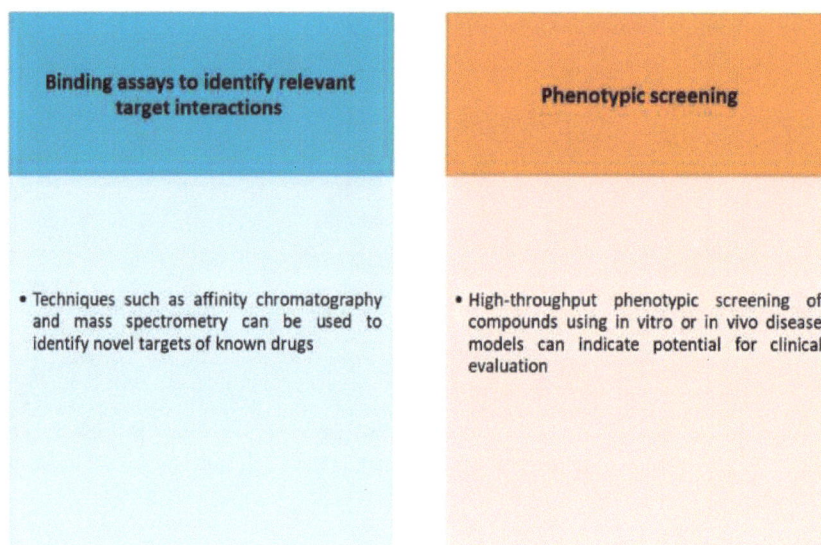

Binding assays to identify relevant target interactions	**Phenotypic screening**
• Techniques such as affinity chromatography and mass spectrometry can be used to identify novel targets of known drugs	• High-throughput phenotypic screening of compounds using in vitro or in vivo disease models can indicate potential for clinical evaluation

Fig. (3). Experimental approaches for identifying repurposing potential of drugs.

Target Associated Screening/Binding Assays to Identify Target Candidate

The targets for the potential drug candidates are identified by proteomics, mass spectrometry, and chromatography techniques [13]. For example, the cellular thermostability assay (CTSA) determines the thermal stabilization of target proteins after binding of high-cellular-affinity compounds. Recently, cellular targets for tyrosine kinase inhibitor (TKI) crizotinib [14] and quinone reductase 2 as an off-target of acetaminophen have been identified [15]. Brehmer *et al.*

performed a study with the help of HeLa cell extract to detect gefitinib protein targets. Mass spectrometry results have shown that gefitinib can interact with 20 distinct protein kinases that can be considered potential targets for gefitinib [13].

Phenotype-based Repurposing

Drug candidates have also been discovered accidentally by phenotypic drug screening methods. New therapeutic molecules can be identified on the basis of *in-vitro* and *in-vivo* modelling or even clinical observations [16, 17]. For example, a compound library is screened using cell lines and based on the cellular response lead compounds are identified, for a specific phenotype along with the mechanisms of action. Further, evaluation of a series of compounds in an array of independent models with the aim of identifying a novel activity among one or more of the tested models fulfils the strategic requirements needed for effective drug repositioning for effective reusability of the medicinal product [18, 19].

In-vitro phenotypic screens require the identification and confirmation of candidates from repositories of known medicines or drug-like molecules. *In vitro* tests can be used to study new diseases based on which repositioning of the drugs can be done. In order to achieve a therapeutic effect over a full concentration range, compounds with a different mechanism of action over the range can also be evaluated [20].

In vivo phenotypical screening is conducted on few selected high-quality drug applicants or compounds rather than on assessing compound libraries. These models can evaluate efficiency, tolerance and safety in general [21]. Genome editing techniques, like CRISPR/Cas-9, are being utilized in combination with preclinical animal studies to model human diseases and perform *in-vivo* screening of old drugs for the phenotypic effects [22].

Clinical Approaches

As most drugs fail in Phase II/III studies, most of the clinical studies do not reach the completion stage. Sometimes, different outcomes are observed during the post-marketing surveillance stage after the drug has reached the market. During this phase, even adverse reactions are observed and on the other hand, cures for diseases, not studied during the clinical trials *i.e.* without any indication on the label can also be discovered. Numerous drugs have already been repurposed as a result of such trials. Some examples include apomorphine, which was originally prescribed for Parkinson's disease but repurposed for erectile dysfunction; drospirenone used as an oral contraceptive and repurposed in hypertension, and dapoxetine which was to be used for analgesia and depression, was later repurposed for hypertension. These are just a few indications of therapeutically repurposed drugs; there are several drugs that have been repurposed for a variety of new indications [23].

Computational Approaches

Computational methods are mainly data-driven; these include the systematic information of data (for instance expression of genes, chemical structure, genotypes or proteomic data, or electronic health records) that lead to the formulation of hypotheses for repurposing of drugs [24]. Computational methods help in identifying drugs, which can be repurposed at reduced costs and time. This strategy allows the collective analysis of data from various sources, including genomic data, and biomedical and pharmacological data to improve the efficiency of drug repositioning [25]. In general, computer approaches are classified as target-based, knowledge-based, signature-based, pathway and target mechanism-based approaches as shown in Fig. (**4**).

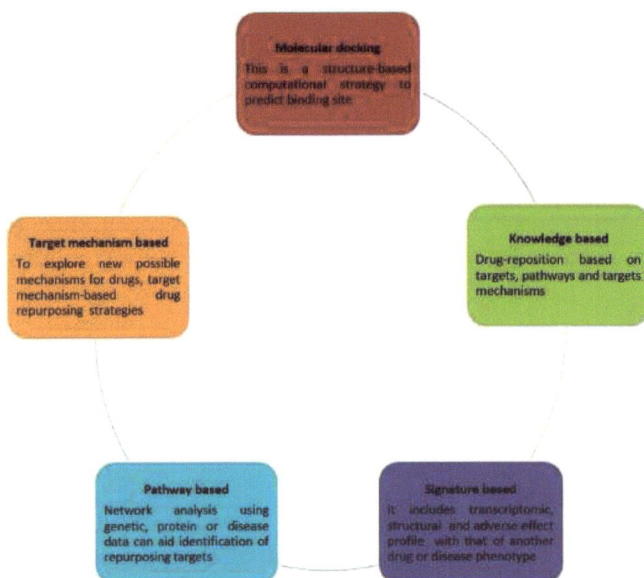

Fig. (4). Different computational approaches can be used as stand-alone or in combination strategies to screen multiple data types to extract valuable insights for hypothesis testing for the repurposing of drugs.

Re-profiling of Drugs Based on Target / Molecular Docking

Target-based drug repurposing involves high throughput and high content screening (HTS/HCS) of pharmacologically active compounds by utilizing proteins and biomarkers, followed by *in silico* ligand or docking based screening of drug compounds [26, 27]. In this screening, no biological or pharmacological information about drug products is incorporated as the screening is blinded. The target-based approach links targets with mechanisms or pathophysiology of disease and thus improves the drug discovery process. The advantage of the targeted approach is that almost all drug molecules of recognized chemical structures can be screened. However, target-based strategies cannot identify unknown mechanisms beyond known objectives [2].

Knowledge-Based

In this drug repurposing approach, models are developed for predicting unidentified targets, bio-markers or disease mechanisms, using drug-related information, such as drug targets, chemical structures, pathways, adverse effects, *etc.* This strategy includes drug reposition based on targets, pathways and targets mechanisms [2].

Signature Based

Signature-based techniques concentrate on identifying genetic factors associated with disease pathophysiologies, such as differentially expressed genes, genetic regulation profiles, and transcription factors. These approaches are elucidating the molecular mechanisms underlying disease pathogenesis. This provides a pathway for the discovery of the drug target mechanisms. Numerous computational tools (such as CMap, GWAS, LINCS, and HGSOC) have been developed to investigate genetic messengers [28].

Pathway Based Repurposing

Protein-protein interactions, cell signalling pathways, and metabolic pathways can all be used to predict how disease and drugs will interact. The best illustration is the information available from the central patient database that can identify the methods of drug repositioning for a specific disease [29].

Target-Mechanism-Based Repurposing

To explore new possible mechanisms for drugs, target mechanism-based drug repurposing combines signalling pathway information using omics data and interacting proteins networks [16]. Such drug-repurposing strategies are stimulated by the growing demand for precision medicine. The advantage of these strategies is that they seek to identify mechanisms not only for disasters but also for drug therapies for specific illnesses [25]. A detailed enumeration of various methodologies of drug repositioning is mentioned in Table **1**.

Table 1. Approaches and methodology for repurposing of drug.

Approaches	Methodology	Specificity	Example	References
Therapy oriented approach	Drug omics data, disease pathway and protein interactions	Signature based bioinformatics, Target based mechanism, Network biology and Systems biology	Sirolimus- acute lymphoblastic leukemia Fasudil-neurodegenerative disorders	[30]
Disease oriented approach	Disease omics data, pathways mechanism	Discoveries of disease mechanism and key targets, disease-specific pathways and gene signatures	Vismodegib- skin cancer Sunitinib, dasatinib- breast cancer	[30]
Drug oriented approach	Phenotyping screening, 3D structures analysis, drug target identifications, clinical trials, adverse effects and FDA approval	Blinded/ Target-based Screening, Cheminformatics, *In silico* screening, ligand-based screening and molecular docking, fragment-based screening, Drug–target prediction and Drug similarity studies	Flurouracil- lung cancer Slidenafil-erectile dysfunction Simavastatin and Ketaconazole- breast cancer	[31]

THERAPEUTIC POTENTIAL OF REPURPOSING OF DRUGS FOR LIFE-THREATENING DISEASES

Drug repurposing or drug re-profiling is the procedure of redevelopment of an existing drug for approval for use as a licensed drug for the different routes of administration with other therapeutic indications [32]. Various drugs and drug categories have been extensively screened with the perspective of repurposing them for urgent and rapid treatment of life-threatening diseases, especially during disease outbreaks or pandemics. The various strategies for the development of repurposed drug encourage the elimination of unnecessary preclinical and clinical protocols and the safety assessment procedures that are required during the development of safe and effective drug for life-threatening diseases [33]. The "Polypharmhacology" aspects of a drug acting on more than one biological target generally led to undesirable side effects due to its off-target activity. As a blessing in disguise, this off-target polypharmacological activity of drugs is being widely utilized for drug repurposing [34, 35]. Government, academics and industries are exploring the repositioning of drugs for different therapeutic purposes. Regulatory agencies of the European Union and United Nation started the initiative known as STAMP which means Safe and Timely Access to Medicines for Patients. Also, drug repurposing programme for supervision and authorization of off-patent medicinal products and launching a workshop with industry, academia and the patient to spread knowledge to support drug repurposing initiatives have been started by the National Institute of Health (NIH). The repositioning of a drug requires computational and experimental data validated for three major criteria: (1) lead candidate selection with all information and indications; (2) theoretical recognition and assessment of drug based on preclinical studies; and (3) safety and efficacy studies of phase II clinical trials [36]. The use of computational approaches for elucidation of chemical structure, genetic expressions through gene mapping pathways especially through genome-wide associated studies (GWAS), proteomic data of the drug candidates, computational molecular docking and clinical analysis have fastened the drug repurposing process [37]. The introduction of the Orphan Drug Act (ODA;1983) for the economic drug development of orphan diseases facilitates rapid approval from the FDA along with funding support to study them for treatment of unknown and rare diseases [38]. After preclinical and clinical analysis, the FDA approves the marketing of the drug with "on-label drug use" extensively for therapeutic purposes. When there is no treatment available for life-threatening diseases, the repurposed drug with proven therapeutic action is known as off-label drugs. Various drugs are repositioned for the treatment of another disease more efficiently than originally reported medications enlisted in Table **2**.

Table 2. A list of repurposed drugs developed for treatment of other disease.

Drug	Original Medication	Repositioned Medication	References
Auranofin	Rheumatoid Arthritis	Metronidazole resistant Giardiasis	[39]
Crizotinib	Anaplastic large-cell lymphoma	Non-small-cell cancer(NSCLC)	[40]
Zidovudine	Anticancer agent	Antiretroviral agent	[3]
Sildenafil	Angina, Chest pain	Erectile myelomas	[41]
Thalidomide	Morning sickness	Multiple Myelomas	[42]
Minoxidil	Hypertension	Androgenic alopecia	[43]
Celecoxib	Pain and inflammation	Familial adenomatous polyps	[44]
Atomoxetine	Parkinson disease	Attention deficit hyperactivity disorder (ADHD)	[45]
Rituximab	Various cancers	Rheumatoid arthritis	[46]

(Table 2) cont.....

Drug	Original Medication	Repositioned Medication	References
Raloxifene	Osteoporosis	Breast cancer	[46]
Fingolimod	Transplant rejection	Multiple sclerosis	[47]
Dapoxetine	Analgesia and depression	Premature ejaculation	[48]
Topiramate	Epilepsy	Obesity	[49]
Ketoconazole	Fungal infections	Cushing Syndrome	[50]
Aspirin	Analgesia	Colorectal cancer	[51]

Advantages of Drug Repurposing

The repurposing of drugs reduces costs, and shortens the timelines and complications, generally associated with the discovery of new drugs.

Cost and Time Minimization

The cost involved in designing a new drug entity restricts the more considerable outcomes of drug discovery. An estimated overview of expenses required for repurposing drugs is estimated to be approximately $1.6 billion which is much lesser than the development of new molecular entities which cost around $12 billion. Moreover, various pharmaceutical companies have reported that $20 billion in annual sales in 2012 were mainly utilized to reposition failed drugs by different pharmaceutical companies. Further, there has been a significant fall in the new drug molecules reaching the market after the year 2000 as reported by Eroom's Law. In contrast, drug repositioning offers lower development time and cost with reduced risk [4]. The biotech drug repositioning companies adopted a business model (Platform, Product, Vertical and Hybrid models) to speed up the development process, shorten the lengthy R&D timeframe, and assessment of drug safety profile and mechanism of action [52].

Accessibility of Information Related to the Drug for Development of Repurposed Drug

The drug-related information like formulation, route of administration, dosing strength, dosage regimen, pharmacokinetic and pharmacodynamics profile, bioavailability data, adverse effects and toxicological data of already approved drugs facilitates the entrance of repurposed drugs in the clinical field with novel therapeutic manifestation. The bioinformatics and cheminformatics databases like Entrez-Gene genetic databases, proteomic database (UniProt), and DrugBank/Drug Central/PubChem are pharmaceutical databases that play a crucial role to build more specific information related to chemical structure and genetic expression for further repositioning of drug [53]. All preclinical, clinical, safety and efficacy data guide the researchers in decision-making to select the orphan drugs with sound scientific basis without any constraints [54].

Dosing Strength and Frequency

The determination of dose accuracy is a complex exercise during drug repositioning that will require substantial development costs, even though API is approved with clear specifications of dosing strength and dosing parameters. The applicability of the therapeutic profile of the drugs for different diseases needs new clinical trials mainly to understand the efficacy of existing drugs to treat life-threatening disorders at suitable dosing strength and frequency. Sildenafil a phosphodiesterase V inhibitor marketed for erectile dysfunction at 25, 50, and 100 mg dosing strength, was repurposed for the treatment of pulmonary hypertension as "Revatio" at dosing strengths 5 and 20 mg [55].

THERAPEUTIC POTENTIAL OF REPURPOSED DRUGS FOR THE TREATMENT OF LIFE-THREATENING DISEASES

Life-threatening diseases are chronically debilitating and caused by pathogens and other factors associated. COVID-19 is a health crisis threatening the world by affecting the respiratory system thus known as severe acute respiratory syndrome coronavirus 2 (SARS-CoV-2) also affects other organs of the body due to oxygen insufficiency. Due to their high complexity and low frequency, important gaps still exist in their prevention, diagnosis, and treatment. Pharmaceutical companies show relatively low interest in orphan drug research and development due to the high cost of investments compared to the low market return of the product due to expensive and time-consuming processes involved in new drug discovery. Therefore, drug repurposing-based approaches appear cost-effective and time-saving strategies for the development of therapeutic opportunities for life-threatening diseases. The understanding of the efficacy and advantages of drug repurposing that has been used earlier for the treatment of various diseases including antiviral infections, tuberculosis, cancer, pulmonary diseases, cardiac diseases and renal dysfunctions has been discussed below.

Tuberculosis

Non-steroidal anti-inflammatory drugs have shown the potential for use as selective anti-mycobacterial for the treatment of tuberculosis. The acid hydrazones and amides of Diclofenac show anti-tubercular activity by inhibiting the incorporation of thymidine and the synthesis of DNA [56]. Mefenamic, meclofenamic acid, indomethacin, and tenoxicam complexes have been found to have anti-tubercular activity against *M. tuberculosis* with <1 µg/mL minimum inhibitory concentration (MIC) values [57]. Celecoxib is a selective COX-2 inhibitor with reported activity against methicillin-resistant *Staphylococcus aureus* and works by inhibiting the bacterial efflux by regulating MDR-1 pump homology in human beings [58]. Ibuprofen has the ability to inhibit inflammatory cytokines mainly tumour necrosis (TNFα) and block the formation of granuloma with minimal threat of liver damage that is generally associated with paracetamol and aspirin [59]. Fluoroquinolones, moxifloxacin and gatifloxacin are broad-spectrum antibiotics that primarily inhibit topoisomerase II and IV, thereby disrupting DNA replication and have shown mycobactericidal activity in phase III clinical trials with pretomanid and pyrazinamide (PaMZ) [60]. Clofazimine is a riminophenazine developed for the treatment of leprosy and has been found beneficial for the treatment of drug-resistant tuberculosis [61]. Biapenem and tebipenem are carbapenem classes of drugs mainly designed to treat infection against *Pseudomonas aeruginosa* and have been repurposed for respiratory pneumonia with MIC_{90} value 2.5-5 ug/ml as anti-tubercular agents with effectiveness against H37Rv *M.tuberculosis* strain with MIC_{90} value 1.25-2.5ug/ml [62]. Ebselen is a seleno-organic compound having antioxidant, anti-inflammatory and anti-atherosclerotic activity and has shown the potential to treat methicillin-resistant tuberculosis. Isoprinosine is an anti-viral immunomodulatory drug that showed *in-vivo* antibacterial activity against *M.tuberculosis* with first-line TB drugs [63].

Moreover, statins reduce the cholesterol level in human macrophages destabilize the membrane and minimize the entrance of pathogens inside macrophages. Simvastatin and pravastatin are examples of cholesterol-lowering agents that have been found to be effective in decreasing bacterial load in TB [64]. Metformin is an oral hypoglycemic agent that mainly targets the host immune response that effectively controls the growth and invasion of *M.tuberculosis* by inhibiting intracellular growth of H37Rv and that of MDR strain in monocyte-derived human macrophages [65].

Cancer

Discovery of new chemotherapeutics by repositioning drugs to overcome multidrug resistance for cancer is being done by docking-based virtual screening (*in-sillico* approach and pharmacophore modelling) for reprofiling of small drug molecules against multidrug-resistant cancer. An anti-schizophrenic drug

"Fluspirilene" has shown the therapeutic potential for the treatment of hepatocellular carcinoma by inhibiting dopamine D2 receptors and blocking the calcium channel, thereby inhibiting the Cyclin-dependent kinase 2 (CDK2) and thus inhibiting cell proliferation and tumour growth [66]. Anti-helminthic drugs Mebendazole and flubendazole are tubulin depolymerization agents, that inhibit tumour growth through inhibition of spindle formation and then apoptosis [67]. Raloxifene is an anti-resorptive agent with the potential to treat cancers by inhibiting the protein-protein IL-6/GP130 interaction [68]. Fenofibrate is a receptor-α agonist (peroxisome proliferator-activated receptor) generally used for dyslipidemia and hypertriglyceridemia, which also inhibits the multiplication of melanoma cells (B16-F10 cells) by downregulation of phosphorylation of Akt and thus suppression of primary tumours' growth [69]. Itraconazole is an antimycotic drug that has also been proven to be efficacious in skin cancer treatment mediated *via* suppressing Wnt, Hedgehog, and PI3K/mTOR signalling pathways [70]. Leflunomide, mainly used for rheumatoid arthritis, acts as an enzyme dihydroorotate dehydrogenase (DHODH) inhibitor which reduces neuroblastoma cell proliferation and induces apoptosis [71]. Some beta-blockers have also shown their potential to treat cancer by inhibiting the pathways involving cyclic adenosine monophosphate (cAMP)-protein kinase that prevents cell proliferation and cell migration in human cancer cell lines, especially in infantile hemangioma (vascular tumor of infancy) [72].

Pulmonary Diseases

Drugs like sildenafil, thalidomide, and raloxifene have been effectively repurposed for the treatment of pulmonary diseases. Slidenafil is a 5 phosphodiesterase (PDE 5) selective inhibitor which has been used for the treatment of angina pectoris and hypertension since 1989 and has also shown a pronounced effect on erectile dysfunction (1998). It was approved for pulmonary arterial hypertension by U.S. Food and Drug Administration (FDA) and Europe, the Middle East, and Africa (EMEA) for treatment of PAH (from 2005 onwards) [73]. Pirfenidone (collagen synthesis inhibitor) is currently approved as an orally active anti-fibrotic molecule for the therapy of idiopathic pulmonary fibrosis (IPF) and reduces radiation-induced fibrosis by inhibiting Type I and III of Collagen Synthesis and mRNA production. Oral pirfenidone has shown good potential for regulating the progression of IPF disease. Preclinical studies with inhaled pirfenidone have shown good antifibrosis activity compared to oral pirfenidone. Pirfenidone has antifibrotic activity and causes reduction of inflammatory cytokines and tumor necrosis factor-alpha (TNF-α), pro-fibrotic growth factors including growth factor-beta (TGF-β), oxidative stress and lipid peroxidation [74].

Cardiac Diseases

Methotrexate is used in the conventional treatment of dyslipidaemia, diabetes and hypertension. Recent studies have shown its potential for treating atherosclerosis and endothelial dysfunction by acetylcholine-mediated and nitroprusside-mediated vasodilation. It also reduces the concentration of IL-6 and TNF-α, thus averting the ICAM-1 and vascular cell adhesion molecule 1, an expression induced by TNF-α that favours the adhesion of leukocytes adhesion to the endothelium in the beginning stages of atherosclerosis [75]. A randomized placebo-controlled study of metformin on the reduction of insulin dependence and carotid artery disease in diabetic patients showed a significant reduction in carotid intima-media thickness, a prolonged therapy of metformin leads to reduced LDL cholesterol, HbA1c levels and estimated glomerular filtration rate (eGFR); further, it has not shown any reduction in the cardiovascular events and HbA1c levels [76].

Antiviral Infections

The viral infections such as Ebola virus, yellow fever virus, Zika virus, Nipah virus, West, Nile virus, dengue virus, SARS-CoV, Middle East respiratory syndrome (MERS-CoV), Influenza virus and human immunodeficiency virus (HIV) have been pestering the mankind every now and then. The surging demand during these viral outbreaks in the absence of vaccines has led to the repositioning of manyexisting drugs. Mycophenolic acid (immunosuppressant) and daptomycin (antibiotic) were the propitious therapeutics in Zika virus infection by restricting viral replication into the host cell. Some antibiotics like novobiocin, niclosamide and temoporfin act as novel zika virus inhibitors targeting NS3/NS2B protease [77]. In contrast, ribavirin and chloroquine were also effective in reducing ZIKV vertical transmission in infected pregnant mice [78]. Statins were also clinically proven for their anti-inflammatory and immunomodulatory effects besides their cardioprotective activity, improving the patient's health in case of severe influenza [79]. Besides this, Nitazoxanide (thiazolide anti-infective) designed to treat parasitic infections, has also shown anti-influenza properties through intracellular trafficking and insertion into the host plasma membrane through selective inhibition of viral glycoprotein HA maturation. Phase IIb/III trial clinical trial (NCT01610245) has shown the efficacy of nitazoxanide in influenza [80]. Recent studies of naproxen analogues showed improved efficacy through blocking NP-RNA and NP-polymerase complexes without inhibiting COX-2 [81].

Remdesivir, a proven potent repurposed drug during the COVID-19 pandemic, was discovered to treat Ebola virus by inhibiting RNA-dependent RNA polymerase (RdRp), but was unable to deliver significant effect in phase III clinical trials. Remdesivir has shown potential anti-viral activity against SARS-CoV, MERS-CoV and SARS-CoV-2. The *in vitro* and *in vivo* preclinical and randomized phase III clinical trials showed a shorter recovery time as compared to other drug treatments in COVID-19. Based on this clinical research, remdesivir got approval from U.S. Food and Drug Administration during COVID-19 outbreak [82]. Conditional approval has also been given by the European medicines agency (EMA) for the treatment of COVID-19 using remdesivir medication in adults and pneumatic adolescents requiring supplemental oxygen delivery for their survival. Some other potential repurposed drugs explored are spironolactone, estradiol, isotretinoin and retinoic acid for down-regulation of ACE_2 receptors. The camostat mesylate, bicalutamide and nafamostat are TMPRSS2 inhibitors also being used as potent agents in COVID-19 treatment.

Similarly, umifenovir and nelfinavir blocks the S protein trimerization thus inhibiting the fusion of the membrane. Studies have demonstrated the activity of dipeptidyl peptidase 4 (DPP4) as a functional receptor for the SARS-CoV-2 (S protein) thereby eliminating the risk of progression of COVID-19. Moreover, antimalarial drugs such as amodiaquine, amiodarone chloroquine, artemisinin hydroxychloroquine, baricitinib, artesunate, niclosamide, chlorpromazine and imatinib restrict the entrance of SARS-CoV-2 inside the host cell by preventing clathrins endocytosis protein, Kinase 1 (adaptor-associated protein) and dynamin.

Favipiravir, sofosbuvir, tenofovir, galidesivir, and clevudine are some antiviral drugs which were reprofiled for reuse in COVID 19 by inhibiting RNA replication. Interferons (alpha interferon and beta interferon) inhibit the replication of the virus and enhance the immune responses to prevent viral infection. Some other therapeutics such as atazanavir, lopinavir, ritonavir, danoprevir, darunavir, and immunosuppressant levamisole are currently used as protease inhibitors for human immunodeficiency virus and acquired immune deficiency syndrome (HIV / AIDS) and have also shown effectiveness by preventing replication of SARS-CoV-2 [82]. Three main categories of repurposed anti-viral agents based on the mechanism and pathophysiology of viral infection have been mentioned in Fig. (**5**).

Repurposed Anti-viral Agents

Direct-acting Repurposed Anti-viral Agents (DARA)	**Multiple Targeting Repurposed Anti-viral**	**Host-Targeting Repurposed Anti-viral Agents**

RNA dependent RNA polymerase inhibitors	**Viral Protease inhibitors**	Dopamine Antagonist-Chlorpromazine	Interferons
Remdesivir	Lopinavir/Ritonavir Rupintrivir	Receptor Tyrosine Kinase inhibitors- sunitinib, Ertotinib	Nitazoxanid
Ribavarin		Lysomotropic Agents-Chloroquine	
Favipiravir		TMPRSS2 inhibitor- Nafamostat Mesylate	
Sofosbuvir		Statins- HMG-CoA Reductase inhibitors	
Galidesivir		Cyclosporine A	

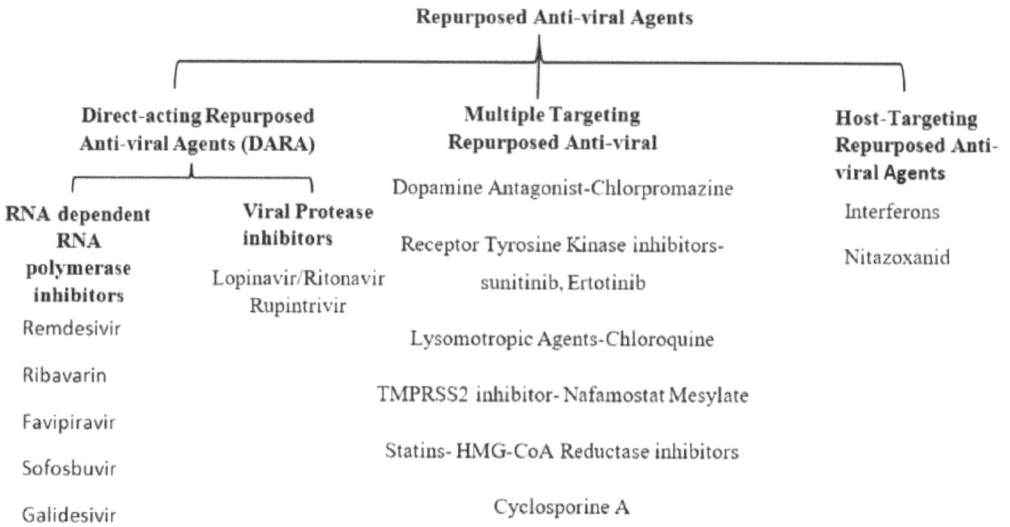

Fig. (5). Classification of Repurposed anti-viral agents with examples based on their mechanism of action [82].

Renal Dysfunction

A potassium agonist of adenosine triphosphate and calcium-sensitizing agent "Levosimendan" has inotropic and vasodilatory effects, and was initially used for acute heart failure. Preclinical research has shown the regenerative potential of levosimendan in ischemia-reperfusion injury by triggering ATP-sensitive potassium channel of mitochondria and nitric oxide (NO) synthase in mice with acute renal failure. It also prevents renal damage from occurring in adult patients during cardiac surgery because of increased blood circulation through vasodilation, renal oxygenation and enhanced glomerular filtration rate (GFR) [83].

Vitamin D maintains calcium hemostasis and is also vital for other systems as well such as immune system, cardiovascular system, renal functions and endothelial systems. The activated vitamin D receptor also regulates the inflammatory response to lipopolysaccharide-induced AKI through the suppression of NF-kb in renal tubules [84]. The antihypertensive effect of GLP-1 and exendin-4 are thought to be due to a decrease in angiotensin II activity, leading to a reduction in renal pathology and other renal impairment events like alterations in sodium homeostasis due to the effect of isoform 3 on the Peripheral Tubules Na^+-H^+ (NHE_3) exchanger [85].

IMPLICATIONS AND IMPORTANCE OF REPURPOSING DRUGS DURING PANDEMIC OUTBREAKS

COVID-19 posed a risk to global health due to the absence of novel agents without clinical efficacy. Reusable drugs have been the only option for SARC-CoV-2 infection. Though vaccine development is underway and few have reached the market as well, it was the repurposing of drugs which played a critical role in controlling the infection. The development of safer and more efficacious drug regimens for patients is a must during any pandemic. The selection of clinically approved drug candidates from the class of antiviral, antimalarial, antineoplastic, antidiabetic, analgesic, and immunomodulatory drugs proved to be beneficial in the management of coronavirus disease. Colchicine, fingolimod, remdesivir, oseltamivir, biorobin, icatibant, Viracept, perphenazine, homoharringtonine, emetine, ribavirin, aloxistatin, valrubicin, almitrine, methylprednisone, famotidine, hesperidin, N4-hydroxycytidine, amprenavir, cromolyn sodium, and antibodies- tocilizumab and sarilumab are list of drugs from the comprehensive list for the treatment of COVID 19 [86]. During the pandemic situation, quick licensing of drugs with minimum available information, depending on the prevalence of the disease and based on data of their biomarkers, benefits and risk assessments and Phase III clinical studies was a great challenge for the health industry. Drugs have been used for COVID 19 treatment, primarily through Emergency FDA authorization, authorization for conditional marketing and approval from the Early Access to Medication Scheme based on less available Phase III clinical data and Phase II results approved for COVID 19 [87]. Therefore, real-life monitoring and evaluation of post-authorization safety and efficacy during a pandemic is required with a conditional license, along with post-marketing surveillance by regulatory authorities.

CONCLUSION

Drug repurposing has emerged as a boon for many chronic disease conditions providing therapeutic potentials within shorter timeframes, lower costs, and fewer risks (the effectiveness and safety of the existing drug against a disease condition are well assessed and approved by the regulatory authorities) surpassing the challenging process of new drug development which requires a huge investment of money and time with no guarantees of return on investment. Drug repurposing has brought new therapeutic scope for many existing drugs against novel/ orphan/ resistant diseases and pandemic outbreaks such as COVID-19. The role of academia, pharmaceutical companies, patient associations, and foundations in the identification of suitable candidates and their preclinical and clinical evaluation becomes a crucial aspect for the emergence of an effective repurposed drug therapy and regime. Furthermore, the challenges faced in existing pre-clinical/clinical studies such as scientific, regulatory aspects, economic aspects, emergency situations, regional limitations of clinical research ethics, involuntary risk burden, regulatory aspects and ethical issues for the development of repurposed drugs have been discussed in chapter 2 (Exploration of Repurposed and Adjuvant Drugs in COVID-19 Patients, as well as Challenges and Ethical Issues Related with Drug Repurposing).

CONSENT FOR PUBLICATION

Not applicable.

CONFLICT OF INTEREST

The author declares no conflict of interest, financial or otherwise.

ACKNOWLEDGEMENTS

Declared none.

REFERENCES

[1] Scherman D, Fetro C. Drug repositioning for rare diseases: Knowledge-based success stories. Therapie 2020; 75(2): 161-7.
[http://dx.doi.org/10.1016/j.therap.2020.02.007] [PMID: 32164975]

[2] Pushpakom S, Iorio F, Eyers PA, *et al.* Drug repurposing: progress, challenges and recommendations. Nat Rev Drug Discov 2019; 18(1): 41-58.
[http://dx.doi.org/10.1038/nrd.2018.168] [PMID: 30310233]

[3] Trivedi J, Mohan M, Byrareddy SN. Drug Repurposing Approaches to Combating Viral Infections. J Clin Med 2020; 9(11): 3777.
[http://dx.doi.org/10.3390/jcm9113777] [PMID: 33238464]

[4] Low ZY, Farouk IA, Lal SK. Drug repositioning: New approaches and future prospects for life-debilitating diseases and the COVID-19 pandemic outbreak. Viruses 2020; 12(9): 1058.
[http://dx.doi.org/10.3390/v12091058] [PMID: 32972027]

[5] Gayathri P, Jaisankar N. Utilization of Data mining Approaches for Prediction of Life Threatening Diseases Survivability. Int J Comput Appl 2012; 41: 51-5.
[http://dx.doi.org/10.5120/5637-8023]

[6] Yella J, Yaddanapudi S, Wang Y, Jegga A. Changing trends in computational drug repositioning. Pharmaceuticals (Basel) 2018; 11(2): 57.
[http://dx.doi.org/10.3390/ph11020057] [PMID: 29874824]

[7] Jourdan JP, Bureau R, Rochais C, Dallemagne P. Drug repositioning: a brief overview. J Pharm Pharmacol 2020; 72(9): 1145-51.
[http://dx.doi.org/10.1111/jphp.13273] [PMID: 32301512]

[8] Pizzorno A, Padey B, Terrier O, Rosa-Calatrava M. Drug Repurposing Approaches for the Treatment of Influenza Viral Infection: Reviving Old Drugs to Fight Against a Long-Lived Enemy. Front Immunol 2019; 10: 531.

[http://dx.doi.org/10.3389/fimmu.2019.00531] [PMID: 30941148]

[9]   Lee WH, Loo CY, Ghadiri M, Leong CR, Young PM, Traini D. The potential to treat lung cancer *via* inhalation of repurposed drugs. Adv Drug Deliv Rev 2018; 133: 107-30.
[http://dx.doi.org/10.1016/j.addr.2018.08.012] [PMID: 30189271]

[10]   Czech T, Lalani R, Oyewumi MO. Delivery Systems as Vital Tools in Drug Repurposing. AAPS PharmSciTech 2019; 20(3): 116.
[http://dx.doi.org/10.1208/s12249-019-1333-z] [PMID: 30771030]

[11]   Cavalla D, Oerton E, Bender A. Drug Repurposing Review. vol. 1–8. Third Edit. Elsevier 2017.

[12]   Cha Y, Erez T, Reynolds IJ, *et al.* Drug repurposing from the perspective of pharmaceutical companies. Br J Pharmacol 2018; 175(2): 168-80.
[http://dx.doi.org/10.1111/bph.13798] [PMID: 28369768]

[13]   Brehmer D, Greff Z, Godl K, *et al.* Cellular targets of gefitinib. Cancer Res 2005; 65(2): 379-82.
[http://dx.doi.org/10.1158/0008-5472.379.65.2] [PMID: 15695376]

[14]   Alshareef A, Zhang HF, Huang YH, *et al.* The use of cellular thermal shift assay (CETSA) to study Crizotinib resistance in ALK-expressing human cancers. Sci Rep 2016; 6(1): 33710.
[http://dx.doi.org/10.1038/srep33710] [PMID: 27641368]

[15]   Miettinen TP, Björklund M. NQO2 is a reactive oxygen species generating off-target for acetaminophen. Mol Pharm 2014; 11(12): 4395-404.
[http://dx.doi.org/10.1021/mp5004866] [PMID: 25313982]

[16]   Jin G, Wong STC. Toward better drug repositioning: prioritizing and integrating existing methods into efficient pipelines. Drug Discov Today 2014; 19(5): 637-44.
[http://dx.doi.org/10.1016/j.drudis.2013.11.005] [PMID: 24239728]

[17]   Kim TW. Drug repositioning approaches for the discovery of new therapeutics for Alzheimer's disease. Neurotherapeutics 2015; 12(1): 132-42.
[http://dx.doi.org/10.1007/s13311-014-0325-7] [PMID: 25549849]

[18]   Lage O, Ramos M, Calisto R, Almeida E, Vasconcelos V, Vicente F. Current screening methodologies in drug discovery for selected human diseases. Mar Drugs 2018; 16(8): 279.
[http://dx.doi.org/10.3390/md16080279] [PMID: 30110923]

[19]   Reaume AG. Drug repurposing through nonhypothesis driven phenotypic screening. Drug Discov Today Ther Strateg 2011; 8(3-4): 85-8.
[http://dx.doi.org/10.1016/j.ddstr.2011.09.007]

[20]   Wilkinson GF, Pritchard K. *In vitro* screening for drug repositioning. SLAS Discov 2015; 20(2): 167-79.
[http://dx.doi.org/10.1177/1087057114563024] [PMID: 25527136]

[21]   Ciallella JR, Reaume AG. *In vivo* phenotypic screening: clinical proof of concept for a drug repositioning approach. Drug Discov Today Technol 2017; 23: 45-52.
[http://dx.doi.org/10.1016/j.ddtec.2017.04.001] [PMID: 28647085]

[22]   Nishimura Y, Hara H. Editorial: Drug repositioning: current advances and future perspectives. Front Pharmacol 2018; 9: 1068.
[http://dx.doi.org/10.3389/fphar.2018.01068] [PMID: 30294274]

[23]   Xue H, Li J, Xie H, Wang Y. Review of drug repositioning approaches and resources. Int J Biol Sci 2018; 14(10): 1232-44.
[http://dx.doi.org/10.7150/ijbs.24612] [PMID: 30123072]

[24]   Hurle MR, Yang L, Xie Q, Rajpal DK, Sanseau P, Agarwal P. Computational drug repositioning: from data to therapeutics. Clin Pharmacol Ther 2013; 93(4): 335-41.
[http://dx.doi.org/10.1038/clpt.2013.1] [PMID: 23443757]

[25]   Park K. A review of computational drug repurposing. Transl Clin Pharmacol 2019; 27(2): 59-63.

[http://dx.doi.org/10.12793/tcp.2019.27.2.59] [PMID: 32055582]

[26]   Swamidass SJ. Mining small-molecule screens to repurpose drugs. Brief Bioinform 2011; 12(4): 327-35.
       [http://dx.doi.org/10.1093/bib/bbr028] [PMID: 21715466]

[27]   Doman TN, McGovern SL, Witherbee BJ, *et al.* Molecular docking and high-throughput screening for novel inhibitors of protein tyrosine phosphatase-1B. J Med Chem 2002; 45(11): 2213-21.
       [http://dx.doi.org/10.1021/jm010548w] [PMID: 12014959]

[28]   Gns HS, Gr S, Murahari M, Krishnamurthy M. An update on Drug Repurposing: Re-written saga of the drug's fate. Biomed Pharmacother 2019; 110: 700-16.
       [http://dx.doi.org/10.1016/j.biopha.2018.11.127] [PMID: 30553197]

[29]   Jadamba E, Shin M. A Systematic Framework for Drug Repositioning from Integrated Omics and Drug Phenotype Profiles Using Pathway-Drug Network. BioMed Res Int 2016; 2016: 1-17.
       [http://dx.doi.org/10.1155/2016/7147039] [PMID: 28127549]

[30]   Sahoo BM, Ravi Kumar BVV, Sruti J, Mahapatra MK, Banik BK, Borah P. Drug Repurposing Strategy (DRS): Emerging Approach to Identify Potential Therapeutics for Treatment of Novel Coronavirus Infection. Front Mol Biosci 2021; 8: 628144.
       [http://dx.doi.org/10.3389/fmolb.2021.628144] [PMID: 33718434]

[31]   Habibi M, Taheri G. Topological network based drug repurposing for coronavirus 2019. PLoS One 2021; 16(7): e0255270.
       [http://dx.doi.org/10.1371/journal.pone.0255270] [PMID: 34324563]

[32]   Padhy BM, Gupta YK. Drug repositioning: Re-investigating existing drugs for new therapeutic indications. J Postgrad Med 2011; 57(2): 153-60.
       [http://dx.doi.org/10.4103/0022-3859.81870] [PMID: 21654146]

[33]   Parvathaneni V, Kulkarni NS, Muth A, Gupta V. Drug repurposing: a promising tool to accelerate the drug discovery process. Drug Discov Today 2019; 24(10): 2076-85.
       [http://dx.doi.org/10.1016/j.drudis.2019.06.014] [PMID: 31238113]

[34]   Reddy AS, Zhang S. Polypharmacology: drug discovery for the future. 2014; 6: 41-7.

[35]   Lavecchia A, Cerchia C. *In silico* methods to address polypharmacology: current status, applications and future perspectives. Drug Discov Today 2016; 21(2): 288-98.
       [http://dx.doi.org/10.1016/j.drudis.2015.12.007] [PMID: 26743596]

[36]   Cichonska A, Rousu J, Aittokallio T. Identification of drug candidates and repurposing opportunities through compound–target interaction networks 2015; 10: 1333-45.
       [http://dx.doi.org/10.1517/17460441.2015.1096926]

[37]   Ko Y. Computational Drug Repositioning: Current Progress and Challenges. Appl Sci (Basel) 2020; 10(15): 5076.
       [http://dx.doi.org/10.3390/app10155076]

[38]   Jegga AG, Zhu C, Aronow BJ. Orphan Diseases. Bioinformatics and Drug Discovery 2012; 16: 287-307.

[39]   Andrade RM, Chaparro JD, Capparelli E, Reed SL. Auranofin is highly efficacious against Toxoplasma gondii *in vitro* and in an *in vivo* experimental model of acute toxoplasmosis. PLoS Negl Trop Dis 2014; 8(7): e2973.
       [http://dx.doi.org/10.1371/journal.pntd.0002973] [PMID: 25079790]

[40]   Bang YJ. The potential for crizotinib in non-small cell lung cancer: a perspective review. Ther Adv Med Oncol 2011; 3(6): 279-91.
       [http://dx.doi.org/10.1177/1758834011419002] [PMID: 22084642]

[41]   Ghofrani HA, Osterloh IH, Grimminger F. Sildenafil: from angina to erectile dysfunction to pulmonary hypertension and beyond. Nat Rev Drug Discov 2006; 5(8): 689-702.

[http://dx.doi.org/10.1038/nrd2030] [PMID: 16883306]

[42] Rahmat M, Sklavenitis Pistofidis R, Ghobrial IM. Repositioning the Repurposed Drug, a Structural Study of Thalidomide Analogs. Hematologist 2019; 16(3): 9556.
[http://dx.doi.org/10.1182/hem.V16.3.9556]

[43] Bryan J. How minoxidil was transformed from an antihypertensive to hair-loss drug. Pharm J 2011; 287: 137-8.

[44] Lynch PM, Ayers GD, Hawk E, *et al.* The safety and efficacy of celecoxib in children with familial adenomatous polyposis. Am J Gastroenterol 2010; 105(6): 1437-43.
[http://dx.doi.org/10.1038/ajg.2009.758] [PMID: 20234350]

[45] Marsh L, Biglan K, Gerstenhaber M, Williams JR. Atomoxetine for the treatment of executive dysfunction in Parkinson's disease: A pilot open-label study. Mov Disord 2009; 24(2): 277-82.
[http://dx.doi.org/10.1002/mds.22307] [PMID: 19025777]

[46] Slimani S, Lukas C, Combe B, Morel J. Rituximab in rheumatoid arthritis and the risk of malignancies: Report from a French cohort. Joint Bone Spine 2011; 78(5): 484-7.
[http://dx.doi.org/10.1016/j.jbspin.2010.11.012] [PMID: 21196130]

[47] Chen W, Chen W, Chen S, Uosef A, Ghobrial RM, Kloc M. Fingolimod (FTY720) prevents chronic rejection of rodent cardiac allografts through inhibition of the RhoA pathway. Transpl Immunol 2021; 65: 101347.
[http://dx.doi.org/10.1016/j.trim.2020.101347] [PMID: 33131698]

[48] McCarty E, Dinsmore W. Dapoxetine: an evidence-based review of its effectiveness in treatment of premature ejaculation. Core Evid 2012; 7: 1-14.
[http://dx.doi.org/10.2147/CE.S13841] [PMID: 22315582]

[49] Kirov G, Tredget J. Add-on topiramate reduces weight in overweight patients with affective disorders: a clinical case series. BMC Psychiatry 2005; 5(1): 19.
[http://dx.doi.org/10.1186/1471-244X-5-19] [PMID: 15817130]

[50] Shirley M. Ketoconazole in Cushing's syndrome: a profile of its use. Drugs Ther Perspect 2021; 37(2): 55-64.
[http://dx.doi.org/10.1007/s40267-020-00799-7]

[51] Chan AT, Giovannucci EL, Meyerhardt JA, Schernhammer ES, Curhan GC, Fuchs CS. Long-term use of aspirin and nonsteroidal anti-inflammatory drugs and risk of colorectal cancer. JAMA 2005; 294(8): 914-23.
[http://dx.doi.org/10.1001/jama.294.8.914] [PMID: 16118381]

[52] Shimasaki C. Understanding Biotechnology Business Models and Managing Risk 2014; 161-74.
[http://dx.doi.org/10.1016/B978-0-12-404730-3.00012-9]

[53] Dhir N, Jain A, Mahendru D, Prakash A, Medhi B. Drug Repurposing and Orphan Disease Therapeutics 2020; 91941.

[54] Pillaiyar T, Meenakshisundaram S, Manickam M, Sankaranarayanan M. A medicinal chemistry perspective of drug repositioning: Recent advances and challenges in drug discovery. Eur J Med Chem 2020; 195: 112275.
[http://dx.doi.org/10.1016/j.ejmech.2020.112275] [PMID: 32283298]

[55] Oprea TI, Overington JP. Computational and practical aspects of drug repositioning. Assay Drug Dev Technol 2015; 13(6): 299-306.
[http://dx.doi.org/10.1089/adt.2015.29011.tiodrrr] [PMID: 26241209]

[56] Maitra A, Bates S, Shaik M, *et al.* Repurposing drugs for treatment of tuberculosis: a role for non-steroidal anti-inflammatory drugs. Br Med Bull 2016; 118(1): 138-48.
[http://dx.doi.org/10.1093/bmb/ldw019] [PMID: 27151954]

[57] Kovala-Demertzi D, Dokorou V, Primikiri A, *et al.* Organotin meclofenamic complexes: Synthesis,

crystal structures and antiproliferative activity of the first complexes of meclofenamic acid – Novel anti-tuberculosis agents. J Inorg Biochem 2009; 103(5): 738-44.
[http://dx.doi.org/10.1016/j.jinorgbio.2009.01.014] [PMID: 19237201]

[58]   Kalle AM, Rizvi A. Inhibition of bacterial multidrug resistance by celecoxib, a cyclooxygenase-2 inhibitor. Antimicrob Agents Chemother 2011; 55(1): 439-42.
[http://dx.doi.org/10.1128/AAC.00735-10] [PMID: 20937780]

[59]   Maitra A, Bates S, Shaik M, *et al.* Repurposing drugs for treatment of tuberculosis: a role for non-steroidal anti-inflammatory drugs. Br Med Bull 2016; 118(1): 138-48.
[http://dx.doi.org/10.1093/bmb/ldw019] [PMID: 27151954]

[60]   Maitra A, Bates S, Kolvekar T, Devarajan PV, Guzman JD, Bhakta S. Repurposing—a ray of hope in tackling extensively drug resistance in tuberculosis. Int J Infect Dis 2015; 32: 50-5.
[http://dx.doi.org/10.1016/j.ijid.2014.12.031] [PMID: 25809756]

[61]   Mirnejad R, Asadi A, Khoshnood S, *et al.* Clofazimine: A useful antibiotic for drug-resistant tuberculosis. Biomed Pharmacother 2018; 105: 1353-9.
[http://dx.doi.org/10.1016/j.biopha.2018.06.023] [PMID: 30021373]

[62]   van Rijn SP, Zuur MA, Anthony R, *et al.* Evaluation of Carbapenems for Treatment of Multi- and Extensively Drug-Resistant *Mycobacterium tuberculosis*. Antimicrob Agents Chemother 2019; 63(2): e01489-18.
[http://dx.doi.org/10.1128/AAC.01489-18] [PMID: 30455232]

[63]   An Q, Li C, Chen Y, Deng Y, Yang T, Luo Y. Repurposed drug candidates for antituberculosis therapy. Eur J Med Chem 2020; 192: 112175.
[http://dx.doi.org/10.1016/j.ejmech.2020.112175] [PMID: 32126450]

[64]   Tahir F, Arif T. Bin, Ahmed J, Shah SR, Khalid M. Anti-tuberculous Effects of Statin Therapy: A Review of Literature. Cureus 2020; 12.

[65]   Naicker N, Sigal A, Naidoo K. Metformin as Host-Directed Therapy for TB Treatment: Scoping Review. Front Microbiol 2020; 11: 435.
[http://dx.doi.org/10.3389/fmicb.2020.00435] [PMID: 32411100]

[66]   XN S, H L, H Y, X L, L L, KS L, *et al. In Silico* Identification and *In Vitro* and *In Vivo* Validation of Anti-Psychotic Drug Fluspirilene as a Potential CDK2 Inhibitor and a Candidate Anti-Cancer Drug. PLoS One 2015; 10: 0132072.

[67]   Guerini AE, Triggiani L, Maddalo M, *et al.* Mebendazole as a Candidate for Drug Repurposing in Oncology: An Extensive Review of Current Literature. Cancers (Basel) 2019; 11(9): 1284.
[http://dx.doi.org/10.3390/cancers11091284] [PMID: 31480477]

[68]   Dinić J, Efferth T, García-Sosa AT, *et al.* Repurposing old drugs to fight multidrug resistant cancers. Drug Resist Updat 2020; 52: 100713.
[http://dx.doi.org/10.1016/j.drup.2020.100713] [PMID: 32615525]

[69]   Cortés H, Reyes-Hernández OD, Alcalá-Alcalá S, *et al.* Repurposing of Drug Candidates for Treatment of Skin Cancer. Front Oncol 2021; 10: 605714.
[http://dx.doi.org/10.3389/fonc.2020.605714] [PMID: 33489912]

[70]   Liang G, Liu M, Wang Q, *et al.* Itraconazole exerts its anti-melanoma effect by suppressing Hedgehog, Wnt, and PI3K/mTOR signaling pathways. Oncotarget 2017; 8(17): 28510-25.
[http://dx.doi.org/10.18632/oncotarget.15324] [PMID: 28212537]

[71]   Zhu S, Yan X, Xiang Z, Ding HF, Cui H. Leflunomide reduces proliferation and induces apoptosis in neuroblastoma cells *in vitro* and *in vivo*. PLoS One 2013; 8(8): e71555.
[http://dx.doi.org/10.1371/journal.pone.0071555] [PMID: 23977077]

[72]   Nguyen H, Pickrell B, Wright T. Beta-blockers as therapy for infantile hemangiomas. Semin Plast Surg 2014; 28(2): 087-90.
[http://dx.doi.org/10.1055/s-0034-1376259] [PMID: 25045334]

[73]   Montani D, Chaumais MC, Savale L, *et al*. Phosphodiesterase type 5 inhibitors in pulmonary arterial hypertension. Adv Ther 2009; 26(9): 813-25.
[http://dx.doi.org/10.1007/s12325-009-0064-z] [PMID: 19768639]

[74]   Ruwanpura SM, Thomas BJ, Bardin PG. Pirfenidone. Am J Respir Cell Mol Biol 2020; 62(4): 413-22.
[http://dx.doi.org/10.1165/rcmb.2019-0328TR] [PMID: 31967851]

[75]   Mangoni AA, Tommasi S, Zinellu A, Sotgia S, Carru C, Piga M, *et al*. Repurposing existing drugs for cardiovascular risk management: a focus on methotrexate. Drugs Context 2018;7:212557.
[http://dx.doi.org/10.7573/dic.212557]

[76]   Schubert M, Hansen S, Leefmann J, Guan K. Repurposing Antidiabetic Drugs for Cardiovascular Disease. Front Physiol 2020; 11: 568632.
[http://dx.doi.org/10.3389/fphys.2020.568632] [PMID: 33041865]

[77]   Munjal A, Khandia R, Dhama K, *et al*. Advances in Developing Therapies to Combat Zika Virus: Current Knowledge and Future Perspectives. Front Microbiol 2017; 8: 1469.
[http://dx.doi.org/10.3389/fmicb.2017.01469] [PMID: 28824594]

[78]   Mercorelli B, Palù G, Loregian A. Drug Repurposing for Viral Infectious Diseases: How Far Are We? Trends Microbiol 2018; 26(10): 865-76.
[http://dx.doi.org/10.1016/j.tim.2018.04.004] [PMID: 29759926]

[79]   Mehrbod P, Omar AR, Hair-Bejo M, Haghani A, Ideris A. Mechanisms of Action and Efficacy of Statins against Influenza. Biomed Res Int 2014; 2014.
[http://dx.doi.org/10.1155/2014/872370]

[80]   Gamiño-Arroyo AE, Guerrero ML, McCarthy S, *et al*. Efficacy and Safety of Nitazoxanide in Addition to Standard of Care for the Treatment of Severe Acute Respiratory Illness. Clin Infect Dis 2019; 69(11): 1903-11.
[http://dx.doi.org/10.1093/cid/ciz100] [PMID: 30753384]

[81]   Sanz-Ezquerro JJ, Fernández Santarén J, Sierra T, *et al*. The PA influenza virus polymerase subunit is a phosphorylated protein. J Gen Virol 1998; 79(Pt 3): 471-8.
[http://dx.doi.org/10.1099/0022-1317-79-3-471] [PMID: 9519825]

[82]   Li X, Peng T. Strategy, Progress, and Challenges of Drug Repurposing for Efficient Antiviral Discovery. Front Pharmacol 2021; 12: 660710.
[http://dx.doi.org/10.3389/fphar.2021.660710] [PMID: 34017257]

[83]   Yilmaz MB, Grossini E, Silva Cardoso JC, *et al*. Renal effects of levosimendan: a consensus report. Cardiovasc Drugs Ther 2013; 27(6): 581-90.
[http://dx.doi.org/10.1007/s10557-013-6485-6] [PMID: 23929366]

[84]   Du J, Jiang S, Hu Z, Tang S, Sun Y, He J, *et al*. Vitamin D receptor activation protects against lipopolysaccharide-induced acute kidney injury through suppression of tubular cell apoptosis. 2019; 316: F1068-77.
[http://dx.doi.org/10.1152/ajprenal.00332.2018]

[85]   Filippatos TD, Elisaf MS. Effects of glucagon-like peptide-1 receptor agonists on renal function. World J Diabetes 2013; 4(5): 190-201.
[http://dx.doi.org/10.4239/wjd.v4.i5.190] [PMID: 24147203]

[86]   Yousefi H, Mashouri L, Okpechi SC, Alahari N, Alahari SK. Repurposing existing drugs for the treatment of COVID-19/SARS-CoV-2 infection: A review describing drug mechanisms of action. Biochem Pharmacol 2021; 183: 114296.
[http://dx.doi.org/10.1016/j.bcp.2020.114296] [PMID: 33191206]

[87]   Starokozhko V, Kallio M, Kumlin Howell Å, *et al*. Strengthening regulatory science in academia: STARS, an EU initiative to bridge the translational gap. Drug Discov Today 2021; 26(2): 283-8.
[http://dx.doi.org/10.1016/j.drudis.2020.10.017] [PMID: 33127567]

CHAPTER 2

Exploration of Repurposed and Adjuvant Drugs in COVID-19 Patients, as well as Challenges and Ethical Issues Related to Drug Repurposing

Malti Dadheech[1] and **Anand Kumar Maurya[1,*]**

[1] *Department of Microbiology, All India Institute of Medical Sciences, Bhopal, India*

Abstract: The Coronavirus Disease (COVID-19), also referred to as Novel Coronavirus Disease, is a contagious viral disease with a high rate of confirmed cases. Therefore, treatment options are urgently needed to fight the deadly virus. Since there is no standard treatment available, it results in increased morbidity and mortality. The development process of a new drug takes years, so it is crucial to focus on repurposed drugs to reduce the severity of this disease. This review aims to describe the regulatory and molecular aspects of repurposed and adjuvant drugs for COVID-19 based on registered clinical trials and online literature. The use of repurposed drugs brings its own ethical issues and challenges. The challenges of the correct interpretation of existing pre-clinical/clinical evidence and the generation of new evidence concerning drug repurposing in COVID-19 and the issues faced by the repurposing community will also be discussed in the review. When drug repurposing is employed in emergency situations, regional limitations of clinical research ethics, involuntary risk burden, regulatory aspects and ethical issues, fairness in resource distribution for repurposed drugs become an issue that requires careful ethical consideration.

Keywords: Adjuvant drugs, COVID-19, Ethical issues, Repurposed drugs.

INTRODUCTION

The pandemic of Coronavirus Disease (COVID-19) caused by Severe Acute Respiratory Syndrome Corona Virus-2 (SARS-CoV2) belongs to the Coronaviridae family of viruses, which is characterized by a high recombination rate that enables it to replicate among animals and humans. Occasionally, recombination in the virus genome within a random host gives rise to a contagious strain, which turns out to be highly pathogenic [1]. The confirmed cases of COVID-19 were heterogeneous and divided into 3 stages; 1) Mild, 2) Severe and 3) Critical cases. Clinical manifestations, such as fever, fatigue and cough, were

* **Corresponding author Anand Kumar Maurya:** Department of Microbiology, All India Institute of Medical Sciences, Bhopal 462020 Madhya Pradesh, India; E-mail:anand.microbiology@aiimsbhopal.edu.in

Tabish Qidwai (Ed.)

the most common in the majority of cases. Others were myalgia, increased levels of aspartate aminotransferase, C-reactive protein, creatine kinase and creatinine, mostly observed in the complicated cases [2].

Since no standard treatment is available, it results in increased morbidity and mortality. Apart from that, a lack of understanding about drug targets and individual perceptions are adding complications to treating the deadly disease. Therefore, therapeutic plans to counteract COVID-19 infection should be devised. It is very important to evolve a comprehensive understanding of how the virus takes over the host during the infection, and apply this understanding towards the development of both repurposed and adjuvant drugs.

The development process of a novel drug is very complicated, highly expensive and needs 10 to 15 years of research. After the production and designing of the drug, it is also important to examine its pharmacokinetics, pharmacodynamics, toxicity and efficacy in cell and animal-based models [3].

Therefore, exploring effective therapeutic agents to combat COVID-19 is essential and urgent [4]. Therefore, it is very crucial to aim at already available anti-viral and adjuvant drugs to reduce the severity of the disease.

Drug repositioning is a process for the identification of new usage for formerly approved therapeutics and is considered a veritably successful approach for drug discovery because it involves less cost and time to find a remedial agent in comparison to the novel drug discovery process [5]. The molecular pathways of these medicines can also be involved in different diseases. According to a study, 75 percent of formerly approved drugs could be repositioned for the treatment of many diseases [6].

Drug repurposing (DR) can ameliorate the recovery rate by decelerating the replication of COVID-19 contagion and also reducing the symptoms. The Intensive Care Units (ICU) could also be relieved from the pressure by syncopating the time spent by the patients in ICU, which makes it an equal possibility for other patients as well to get the services [7]. Hence, the fastest process to manage the pandemic situation is to repurpose the formerly approved drugs that have been used with a known safety profile [3, 9].

Adjuvant drugs are non-habit-forming, non-opioid medications that can be used as "add-on therapy" to help in the treatment of pain (https://nwapain.com/adjuvant-medications). Frequently used supplements, such as Vitamin-C and zinc, have been reported to decrease the time and seriousness of viral diseases by raising the immune response [8]. The proof supporting supplement therapy as a treatment for infections caused by a virus is very restricted [9]. In the COVID-19 era and rapidly increasing death rates, there is a desperate need for successful treatment options; whether these supplement molecules could be helpful for the patients infected with the SARS-CoV2 virus is a research question worth assessing [9].

The potential repurposing therapeutics to treat the SARS-CoV-2 infection are anti-malarial, anti-viral, anti-biotic, immunosuppressants, monoclonal antibodies, nti-anthelmintic, ngiotensin-converting enzyme inhibitors, Kinase inhibitors, anti-bacterial, anti-diabetic drugs, anti-tumoral, interferons and others [8].

Potential candidates for adjuvant therapy for SARS-CoV-2 are Resveratrol, stilbene-bases natural compounds, N. Sativa (Black seed), Zinc, HMG CoA reductase inhibitors (statins), Melatonin, Indomethacin, Iron chelators, Vitamin-D, Vitamin-C and others [10].

POTENTIAL CANDIDATES FOR ADJUVANT THERAPY

The potential candidates for adjuvant therapy are summarized below in Table **1**.

Vitamin D

Vitamin D (Vit-D) shows antimicrobial and immunomodulatory activities and is also used as an adjuvant therapy to reduce the consequences of different conditions [11]. According to various studies, people with Vit-D deficiency have a greater chance of developing respiratory infections [12]. When the skin is exposed to UVB rays during the summer season, Vit-D is produced as a secosteroid [13]. COVID-19 severity can be very high in patients with hypovitaminosis (Skin produces less Vit-D in skin) [14]. Research shows that Vit-D plays an important role in balancing the renin-angiotensin system (RAS) and the reduction of lung damage [14]. From a molecular perspective, Vit-D accelerates the differentiation of monocytes into macrophages, enhances leukocyte recruitment and chemotaxis and increases the antimicrobial activity of the innate immune system [15]. It also promotes the production and secretion of defensins and cathelicidin and reinforces the barrier function of different organs [16].

Many studies obtained heterogeneous data by analyzing the role of Vit-D supplementation as treatment and preventive therapy of respiratory infections [16]. However, in most of the clinical trials on paediatric cases, the intervention consists of the administration of 400-1200 IU of Vit-D daily [17]. Therefore, supplements within this range can be advised for COVID-19 prevention.

Stilbenoids

Many plants produce stilbenoids as natural phenolic compounds. They are produced by plants in response to bacterial and fungal toxins and UV radiation [18]. The most widely studied and prominent stilbenoid is resveratrol due to its antioxidative [19], antitumoral, anti-viral, life span extension and anti-inflammatory activities.

The analogues of stilbenoids could be a prospected supplier of the human ACE2 (hACE2) receptor and spike protein of SARS-CoV-2. In a study, a crystal structure of SARS-CoV-2 spike (S)-protein with hACE2 complex revealed the importance of stilbenoid as an appropriate aim to develop strong curatives. These curatives will be very helpful in the destruction of S protein and hACE2 interface.

Considering that the novel coronavirus has become a global pandemic, repurposing already available plant-based and synthetic drugs, is prospected to be of great benefit to eliminate and control the COVID-19 disease [20].

Curcumin

In various studies, therapeutic effects of natural compounds such as natural polyphenol and curcumin have been reported, including potential antioxidant, anti-inflammatory, anti-viral, chemotherapeutic, and antibacterial properties [21]. The clinical studies have investigated the effects of nano-encapsulated curcumin in patients infected with COVID-19. A significant reduction in clinical symptoms of coronavirus was observed in the mild and severe disease patient group treated with nano curcumin [22]. A study done by Wen *et al.* (2007) observed curcumin's anti-viral activity in Vero-E6 cells against the SARS-CoV2 virus, and at some concentration, it could also hamper the replication of the virus [23]. Many scientists are using the *in-silico* models to estimate the capability against SARS-CoV-2 receptors and binding proteins [24].

Zinc (Zn)

Zinc is found in human's intra-cellular compartments. The distribution of Zinc varies in every organelle. The Zn level in the nucleus is 30–40%, cytosol and other cell organelles and specialized vesicles contain 50% of the Zn, and the remaining is bound with the cell membrane proteins [25]. Plasma Zn level in humans ranges b/w 10–18 mol/Litre [26]. Trace element Zinc is important for the functioning and development of the immune system [27]. Zn deficiency results in dysfunction and an altered number of immune system cells [28].

Several studies have proved the significance of Zn for the growth and function of the immune system [29, 30]. The deficiency of Zn results in dysfunction and an altered number of immune cells. The suboptimal zinc level has escalated chances for autoimmune disorders, cancer and infectious diseases [31, 32]. Elderly persons and subjects with autoimmune and inflammatory diseases have a higher risk of Zn deficiency [33, 34]. According to WHO, at least 1/3 of the entire world population is affected by the deficiency of Zn [35]. Over 16% of respiratory infections are caused by Zn deficiency [36]. Therefore, Zn is beneficial to cure the severe progression of SARS-CoV2 infection.

Over 17% of the world population is predicted to be deficient for Zn, and approximately 20% of diets contain an insufficient quantity of Zn to meet minimum health requirements. The Zn deficiency is the highest in Central America, South America, Sub-Saharan and South-East Asia region. Marginal deficiencies of Zn are also prevalent in developed regions [36].

Headaches, rough skin, mental lethargy, irritability, slow tissue repair, recurrent infections, mental lethargy, and reduced lean body mass are the clinical presentation related to mild and moderate zinc deficiency [37].

According to a recent non-systematic review, Zn has the capability to prevent lung injury induced by the ventilator, modulate anti-viral immunity, improve mucociliary clearance and reduce inflammation [37].

Many studies have illustrated that Zn may inhibit the angiotensin-converting enzyme 2 (ACE2) activity and hamper the replication of RNA polymerase [38]. Another repercussion due to deficiency of Zn comprises an elevated risk of vitamin-A deficiency that is also crucial for immune functions [39]. The role of zinc as a supportive therapy gives anti-viral as well as immunological support. Zn also plays a crucial role in coagulation and haemostatic modulation acting as an effector of fibrinolysis and anticoagulation [40, 41]. Zinc intake improves neurological recovery after a brain stroke. Zinc intake and its effectiveness in the treatment and prevention of COVID-19 are still to be evaluated [37].

The direct effect of Zn on COVID-19 is not well studied, but its anti-viral activity, immunomodulatory effect, and its potential to control the inflammatory response [38, 42, 43]. The potential process by which Zn might be beneficial in the prevention and treatment of COVID-19 is based on the former studies and other common respiratory viral infections. Zn has been found to increase and refine ciliary beat frequency. Zn is observed as a membrane stabilizer and also as an aid to keep up the integrity of the cytoskeletal. Zn inhibits the RdRp to block the multiplication of the virus and stop the virus entry. SIRT-1-induced ACE-2 receptor expression is reduced by Zn. Zn helps enhance the level of IFN-α and the synthesis of anti-viral proteins, such as protein kinase RNA and ribonuclease, which degrades the viral RNA [44, 45]. Zn also has antioxidant activity and decreases the production of reactive oxygen species and reactive nitrogen species [46]. Zn also has been found to raise natural killer cells, cytotoxic T cells activity, signalling B Cell Receptor, and antibody production and also control regulatory T-cell functions [47, 48].

Overall, the above-mentioned finding build up the truth that Zn is necessary to shield a person from viral infection. A daily Zn uptake of up to 40 mg is recommended to conquer the COVID-19 infection [49].

In COVID-19 patients, there is a decrease in the sufficient secretion of type I and II interferons [50]. The supplementation of Zn can enhance its anti-viral activity by JAK/STAT1 signalling and reconstruct its expression by leukocytes as detected for rhinovirus-infected cells [51, 52]. Recently, Ziegler *et al.* addressed that COVID-19 might benefit from interferon-dependent ACE2 expression [53]. The effect of Zn supplementation needs to be further estimated [27].

Melatonin

A bioactive molecule referred to as melatonin (N-acetyl-5-methoxytryptamine) has some useful activity to cure delirium, respiratory diseases, sleep disorders and infectious agent (viral) infections [54]. Antecedently reported studies had illustrated the effect of melatonin on decreasing bacterial, viral and radiation-induced acute respiratory stress [55 - 57]. The theory for the use of melatonin in viral diseases is supported by Reiter *et al.* [58]. Melatonin can potentially attenuate COVID-19 infection by its immune enhancing features such as anti-oxidation, anti-inflammation activities [59 - 61] and also weakens the oxidative stress and severe inflammatory responses caused by COVID-19 infection. Melatonin inhibits the protein calmodulin and indirectly hampers the SARS-CoV-2 and ACE-2 binding [62].

The RNA of the virus is firstly released into the cytoplasm of host, and then the translation of the viral genome takes place to form new particles of the virus [63].

Melatonin inhibits Angiotensin-2 and promotes the activity of angiotensin 1-7 [64]. There is no current data on clinical trials to utilize melatonin as a medication against the SARS CoV-2 infection. Nevertheless, two randomized, double blind clinical trials data were found in which melatonin was used as 5 mg. twice a day for seven consecutive days in the form of oral capsule and 5 mg per kilogram as per bodyweight every six hours for seven days as intravenous dose [65, 66]. Additionally, the website clinicaltrials.gov mentions six ongoing clinical trials (NCT04784754, NCT04409522, NCT04530539, NCT04470297, NCT04474483 and NCT04353128) which are utilizing melatonin as a treatment in patients infected with COVID-19 [67 - 72].

Although the above mentioned trials will give insights into the benefits of melatonin in the treatment of COVID-19 but they do not concentrate on the treatment in the beginning of diagnosis. Due to the pandemic urgency and melatonin safety profile, it can be used before conducting clinical trials for the COVID-19 treatment [63].

Iron Chelators

There are a number of studies which shows evidence with respect the anti-viral activity of iron chelators. Lectoferrin is a natural iron chelator that exerts anti-inflammatory and immunomodulatory activity. Iron chelators have high therapeutic value against COVID-19 due to its binding with receptors utilized by corona virus and thereby blocking their entry into the host cell [73].

COVID-19 attacks hemoglobin, dissociates por-phyrins from iron and releases iron. Therefore haemoglobin hampers its delivery to body organs by losing its capacity capacity leading to into multi organ failure. Released irons cause oxidative damage to multiple organs. These points dictate enhanced storage and uptake of iron-binding proteins which results in increased concentration of ferritin in COVID patients. The surge in iron loads to an increase in blood viscocity with circulatory thrombosis. This may cause death in some patients. Iron chelators effective against COVID-19 are lectoferrin, deferoxamine, deferiprone, and deferasirox. Thus, we can think about iron chelators as a useful adjuvant therapy in treating the COVID-19 as they alleviate inflammation and prevent corona virus and host receptor binding [73].

Vitamin C

Ascorbic acid is very easily available along with other necessary adjuvant drugs that patients generally take as therapeutics. Vitamin C plays an essential role in immune response as an antioxidant. There is lack of evidence which recommend that the enhanced dose of Vitamin-C may decrease the severity of clinical manifestations. Nevertheless, part of Vitamin-C in diminishing the manifestation and recovering the patients infected with COVID-19 is undetermined [18].

Table 1. Potential candidates for adjuvant therapy against SARS CoV-2.

Pharmacological Class	Drug	Mechanism Of Action
Immunomidulatory	Vitamin-D	Promotes the T-Reg lymphocytes cells efficiency, suppresses the cytokine storm and enhances the cytokine production by T- Helper cells.

(Table 1) cont.....

Pharmacological Class	Drug	Mechanism Of Action
Anti-viral Anti-Inflammatory Immunomodulatory	Stillbenoides	Promotes the cell proliferation, hACE2 receptor complex inhibition, activates the ERK1/2 signalling, enhances the SIR1 signalling, and disrupts S-protein of the SARS CoV-2.
Anti-viral Anti-Inflammatory Immunomodulatory	Curcumin	Binds to viral attachment sites and S protein to hinder the entry of SARS-CoV2.
Anti-viral Anti-Inflammatory Immunomodulatory	Zinc (Zn)	Enhances the immunity, blocks the entry of SARS-CoV-2 into pneumocytes, inhibits recombinant SARS-CoV RdRp activity.
Anti-Inflammation and Immunomodulatory	Melatonin	Influences the T helper cells, T cytotoxic cells, neutrophils and B cells through melatonin receptors on membrane and regulates the cytokine release and production.
Anti-Inflammatory Immunomodulatory	Iron chelators	It decreases the endothelial and IL-6.
Immunomodulatory	Ascorbic acid (Vitamin-C)	It clears the Reactive Oxygen Species related cellular toxicity.

The potential repurposed therapeutic candidates treat the SARCCoV2 infection are summarized below in Table **2**.

Table 2. Potential candidates for repurposed drugs for SARS CoV-2.

Pharmacological Class	Drug	Mechanism of Action
Inhibitors of Kinase	Baricitinib	Reduces endocytosis of SARS-CoV2 Employs anti-viral effects by showing affinity for AP2-associated protein AAK1.
	Imatinib	Assembles in lysosome Performs lysosomal alkalization for virus and host cell fusion.
Antibacterials	Doxycycline	It is needed for virus and host cell fusion.
-		Chelate the matrix metalloproteinases and inhibit the virus replication.
Antidiabetic drugs	Dapagliflozin	It reduces the oxygen consumption and lactate level in tissues.
-	Linagliptin, sitagliptin	They inhibit DPP4.
Anti-malarials Anti-inflammatory	Artemisinin/artesunate	It has endocytosis inhibition mechanism.
-	Atovaquone	It targets the viral RdRp.

(Table 2) cont.....

Pharmacological Class	Drug	Mechanism of Action
-	Chloroquine, hydroxychloroquine	It counteracts the replication of virus.
-	Mefloquine	It inhibits the replication of SARS-CoV-2.
Antitumorals	Plitidepsin	Destructs the multiplication of SARS-CoV-2.
-	Selinexor	Inhibits the replication of SARS-CoV-2.
Anti-virals	Atazanavir, danoprevir, darunavir	Potential inhibitor of SARS-CoV-2 protease.
-	Clevudine	Acts as a potential inhibitor of RdRp.
-	Daclatasvir	It affects the virion and viral RNA replication assembly.
-	Emtricitabine	It could have an effect on virus infection.
-	Favipiravir, galidesivir	Inhibit RdRp protein of the virus.
-	Lopinavir/ritonavir	Blocks PL2pro and 3CLpro proteases.
-	Nelfinavir	It inhibits the fusion of membrane.
-	Nitazoxanide	An intracellular protein factor 2-alpha is increased which shows anti-viral activity.
-	Oseltamivir	Hinders the viral replication and release of virion.
-	Remdesivir	It could inhibit the RNA synthesis of SARS-Co--2.
-	Ribavirin	It could inhibit SARS-CoV-2 replication.
-	Sofosbuvir	It is a chain terminator for SARS-CoV-2 RNA polymerase. In human brain organoids, it protects from SARS-CoV-2-induced cell death.
-	Tenofovir alafenamide	It could inhibit SARS-CoV-2 RdRp.
-	Umifenovir	Blocks the trimerization of S protein.
Immunosuppressants	Cyclosporine	Blocks the replication of virus and transcription of cytokines.
-	Leflunomide	Studies have shown its effect against SARS-Co--2.
-	Sirolimus	Blocks the release of virion and expression of viral protein.
-	Tacrolimus	Inhibits the SARS-CoV-2 replication
Interferons	Alpha and beta interferons	They inhibit virus replication and support immune response to clear the virus infection.
-	Peginterferon lambda-1A	It inhibits viral replication.
Other	Amiodarone	Affects the cell activity by decreasing the internal acidity of lysosomes and endosomes which is important for viral entry.

(Table 2) cont.....

Pharmacological Class	Drug	Mechanism of Action
-	Bicalutamide, bromhexine, camostat mesilate, nafamostat	Inhibition of the enzyme TMPRSS2 which facilitates cell penetration of SARS-CoV-2.
-	Chlorpromazine	Hampers the encocytosis of clatrine-mediate
-	Estradiol patch	It causes the down-regulation of the ACE2 receptors in kidneys.
-	Famotidine	It could bind with the papain-like protease and hampers the translation of SARS-CoV-2
-	Isotretinoin, retinoic acid	Inhibits the protease and enhances CD4 counts.
-	Ivermectin	Hinders the SARS-CoV-2 virus replication.
-	Niclosamide	S-Phase kinase associated protein 2 is inhibited by this drug.
-	Spironolactone	Causes the reduction of ACE-2 receptor on lung-cell surfaces.
-	Verapamil	It blocks ion channels.

CHALLENGES RELATED TO DRUG REPURPOSING

The use of repurposed drugs brings its own drawbacks and challenges (Fig. **1**).

Limited Repository of Drugs

This challenge arises largely due to the high attrition rate in designing, approval, and development process of the drug [74]. According to a study conducted by Darrow *et al.* (2020) [75], from the year 2010 to 2018, out of hundreds of applications received for drug candidature, only an average of 41 therapeutics per annum were approved by the FDA. This very slow acceptance and high attrition rate are because of the very strict assessment which is important to make sure the efficacy and safety of the drug. Due to a very few number of new drugs approved every year, drug repositioning studies can be more challenging due to the shortage of noval drugs to be repurposed [75].

Limited Efficacy of Repurposed Drugs

The effectiveness of the repurposed drug towards its new target is not powerful as the primary target [76]. So the molecular variations would frequently have to be executed in order to enhance the drug efficacy against the drug target for successful drug repurposing. As a consequence, numerous projects ends up with drug repurposing regarding a target associated with the same class as its initial target. This results into a restricted scope of diseases for which drug repurposing can be carried out to discover therapeutic agents.

Moreover, for obtaining maximized drug efficiency, repositioned drugs may be required which further require clinical as well as pharmaceutical proficiency for achieving correct localized drug delivery. Due to ever-changing scientific data on COVID-19 pandemic, finalizing novel drug designing, formulation and delivery are challenging [77].

Regulatory and Patent Considerations

There are many intellectual and legal property aspects associated with the new use of formerly available drugs. Firstly, some of the legislative assemblies cut off the patent for further use of medicines. Secondly, in various countries, clinicians are not bound to prescribe therapeutics outside of their indicated use. This is named as "off-label" use. This off-label use of the drug is often disapproved by the Regulatory Agencies. For drugs with non-registered use, a patent can be acquired but law enforcement could become a concern if the new use makes use of existing strengths and dosage forms. Thirdly, critical barriers in stimulating drug repositioning, as they have a great influence on the potential benefit expected by the product [77, 78].

The uses of repurposed have been presented in many research articles or in health care practices. Although the patentee may not have proved the work through already available research knowledge, clinical trials of the repurposed drugs may restrict the capability to get the patent protection unless they can somehow modify their patent claims over the information that is already accessible in the public domain. The patentee also needed to present the data illustrating that the drug is a reliable treatment for the novel repurposed use.

The off-label use of the drug is often disapproved by Regulatory Agencies, so a novel method-of-use patent can be approved for these drugs. However, law enforceability can become a critical issue here if generic drugs are used for repurposed indications. The maker of the generic drug can also tag their product for the non-patented use known as 'skinny labelling' [79]. They do not support the use of patented indication in any different way. It will be very tough to claim that they are offending the novel method-of-use patent. By knowing this scheme, it can be much harder to restrict the off-label usage for the newly patented repurposed indication [77, 80].

In 2015, the parliament of United Kingdom stressed upon the fact that the selling of the repositioned drug in the market has been a challenge [3]. A bill known as off-label drugs bill 2015-2016 was introduced in the parliament to be used for factors out of the scope of initial patent, but the same failed to be passed in the assembly [81]. Again in 2017, Medical Research Charities Association (MRCA) in coordination with National Institute for Health and Care Excellence (NICE) published a report for the use of repurposed drugs in the UK. This report included all possibilities in which the sponsors can work with MRCA for licensing and provide financial incentive for the same [82, 83]. In the USA institutions like OPEN ACT provided added 6 months exclusivity to the algidity of the patent in which repurposed drugs will be used for a rare disease. Obtaining exclusive market approval in certain regions and developing new formulations can be other methods for enhancing patentability [81].

Accessibility of Data and Compound

As far as drug discovery is concerned, open source model is gaining popularity but still the clinical trials data are restricted for public access up to a large extent [84]. Actions like data mining, manipulation and integration are not feasible on certain type of data or mostly they are presented in a non standardised format [81]. For enhancing the accuracy of data analysis, integration of all types of raw data has become computationally demanding [85].

Moreover a stored drug could be considered as an idle capital or a postponed chance, some pharma companies are less inclined than others to release the constituents (*e.g.* failed drugs) to branch the possible applications of their compound collections, which could pose a fundamental barrier to drug repurposing prospects if a potential repurposed indication falls outside the organization's core disease area.

Flexible and friendly administrative rules are required for a better crowd response by small players. More emphasis should be on transfer of materials and documented formalities [86].

Other issues might also arise with compound availability of running pharmaceutical constituents.

Getting a trustworthy vendor may result to be a challenging issue [86].

Uncertainty of Space for Repurposing Drugs

It is certainly possible that the possibilities of drug repurposing may get exhausted due to the large number of movements organised. The world is facing ever increasing cases of new diseases every day, suitable associates for these therapeutic drugs are very less in numbers. This has also resulted in the increased possibility of exhaustion of space for these repurposed drugs.

For *e.g.*, several high-throughput screenings for the identification of repurposed drugs for trypanosoma with possible implementation as treatment for Chagas disease have been reported [87 - 91]. This has compromised the experimental accuracy of various screenings because of specific drug targets. The need is to redirect the plans of action towards untouched issues. Examining drug combinations could improve the scope of drug repurposing, for *e.g.* Nifurtimoxeflornithine strategy is used for the second stage trypanosomiasis found in Africa [92]. Other tools which can be effective in expanding the scope of drug repurposing are precision and system medicines. Their execution on ground will again require a conscious effort from all the stake holders trying to make it possible.

Intellectual Property and Economic Considerations

The inducement of drug repurposing may get marginalized due to some legal issues. This directly or indirectly hampers the patenting process of these generic drugs. Some of the national legislations are promptly responsible for impeding the sanctions for these drugs in a large way. Due to such organisations, a large number of potential repositioned drugs so far have been reported for their usage in the market, exposing their unauthorised use.

For these repurposed drugs, a fresh patent can be obtained but their implementation will become an issue in the market if it uses already existing usage patterns of other medicines [81]. A solution to this issue can be some new formulations for these non marketed strengths. Using the same strategy will most probably be unfruitful. Some regions like the European Union and USA provide complete implementation strategy to the originator including data protection for a certain period [81].

Presently, certain Pharmaceutical Companies have started realizing the benefit of these generic medicines and have started digging outside their area of the present occupation. They have also started certain mutual liaisons with small and medium sized biotech firms and other academic institutions, for *e.g.* Astra Zeneca Open Innovation Platform [93]. Some other institutes are the Centre for excellence for experimental drug discovery, at GlaxoSmithKline, Bayer's Grant 4 Indications initiative and Centre for Therapeutic Innovation at Pfizer. Some challenges are also being faced due to repurposed indications being out of the organisational core area or due to the termination of compound's development. This causes the absence of an active project for research development [93]. The issue can be addressed by involving external sources for supply of drugs in collaboration with manufacturing agencies. Finding alternate funding organisations will also be the need of the hour for better repurposing especially for compounds which target unique mechanisms. Moreover, most of these compounds are active in developmental phases. They are involved in certain types of risks to proprietary rights, and if disclosed, may raise concerns with respect to this subject [94].

Another limitation for these repurposed drugs is the non-existence of well defined guidelines for regulation. At present, the utilisation of repurposed drugs for human use is still a big challenge. There is always a risk involved with the personnel's being a part of repurposing because of a failed indication failed indication [95]. A branched programme for development can be a better option as it evaluates several indications simultaneously. There is no surety of economic returns for a pharmaceutical company, when involved in repurposing. The shortage of funding agencies is again a challenge for the drugs. Other limitations involved are technical and legal requirements which hold intellectual property rights which are more difficult to overcome [96]. Another practical issue is developing a resistant microbe for drugs used in case of a variety of diseases. Since the drugs were manufactured for a selective disease in nature, their applicability as repurposed drugs is uncertain and limited as it involves a different kind of disease altogether [86].

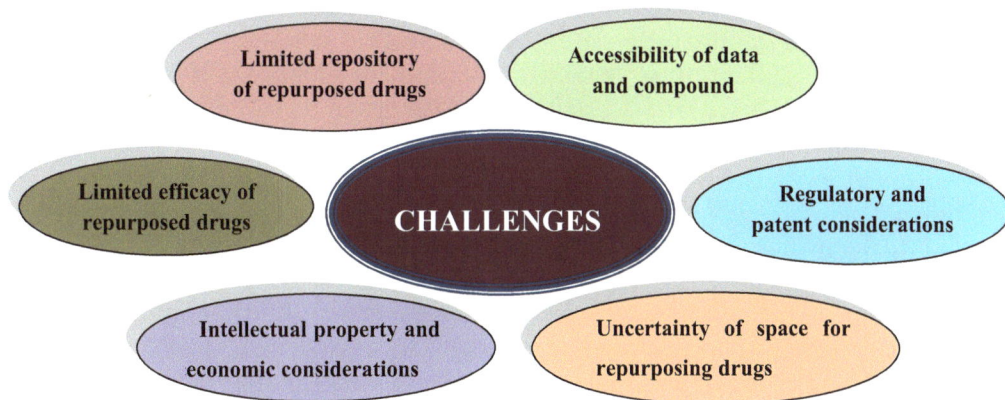

Fig. (1). This figure is demonstrating challenges related to drug repurposing.

ETHICAL ISSUES RELATED TO DRUG REPURPOSING

An article by Emanuel *et al.* [97], delineated 7 requirements that provided a systematic framework to determine whether clinical research and trials are ethical. These 7 were independent review, scientific validity, fair subject selection, value, favourable risk benefit ratio, informed consent and respect for potential and enrolled subjects. Clinical research that violated any of these 7 requirements would be unethical.

While repurposing of drugs, there is an impact on certain group of people. The rapidly increasing cases of COVID-19 raised an immediate demand for the therapeutics and that is how the option of repositioned or repurposed drugs started taking place for this deadly disease. Nevertheless, no studies resolved the issue of repurposing of drugs in the pandemic era, taking into account the ethical and social complications [7].

Regional Limitations of Clinical Research Ethics During Emergency Situations

Region wise restrictions of medical research ethics and exclusive evidence for Original Indication (OI) in the time of crisis like pandemic are under exploitation. The drugs provide a greater efficiency for the OI than for the New Indication (NI) due to the Randomized Controlled Trials (RCTs) organized for the OI. These trials are well-designed and use very detailed scrutiny using the global data as the tools with assured results on longevity [98].

Secondly, the foundation for extensive use of therapeutics for NI is only based on the early stages of the pandemic. Sequencing indications with limited medical proof in this manner is an outlier to the fundamentals of evidence-based therapeutics and is scientifically illogical. There is a necessity of strict ethical reviews for the organization of scientific and ethical precision, but this is not a practical solution, particularly in an emergency situation. There are minimum possibilities for research to be well designed in case of extreme emergencies. Drug discoveries and developments are also very less probable to be fully developed. Therefore due to lack of evidences, the evaluation of drug efficiency becomes difficult [99].

When ethical and scientific backing are missing, drug repurposing turns into a simple off-label product. In case of emergency, if the assessment of Institutional Review Board (IRB) were workable for drug repositioning, the local restrictions of the IRB would be having certain problems. For example, the choice to approve the study at one facility totally depends on the other. While planning for a wider area or the entire country, there would be inevitable problems with resource distribution.

Another example is that IRB verdict verdict could be made on the basis of facility-dependent differences which can create a biased statement in which few patients are prescribed to take the treatment, whereas others are not prescribed. Consequently, for the use of drug repurposing in alarming conditions, simply authorizing the IRB to take the decisions at each facility may not get fair resource distribution at the macro level of public health [99].

Fairness in Resource Distribution for Repurposed Drugs in Emergency Situations

In the COVID-19 pandemic situation or any other emergency situation, there is a concern that requires ethical inspection that is fair distribution of the resources between the NI and OI patients. Emanuel *et al.* reported ethical issues of granting medical resources for COVID-19 [100]. However, in terms of medical resource distribution in alarming conditions, the issue is not the allocation among patients infected with COVID-19, but rather allocation between patients infected with COVID-19 and those infected with other diseases. For examination of the ethics for resource distribution, there is a requirement of a more macroscopic perspective.

As per a case report from Japan, a patient inhaled asthma steroid as the OI which was found to be beneficial against COVID-19 [101]. The pharma enterprise in Japan distributing the drug got subsequently flooded with a number of requests from various institutions and pharmacies related to that medicine. The results indicated they desired to ignore a situation in which the supply needed by existing asthma patients was not enough. This issue came into existence in synchronisation with the DR of the ciclesonide drug to cure COVID-19 [102]. The distribution of these medications according to the patient requirement became hard to manage in few geographical areas of Japan. Later, the Association for Infectious Diseases (Japan) issued a statement about "non applicability" to stop COVID-19 [99].

Subsequently, scarcities of Bacillus Calmette-Guérin (BCG) vaccine were observed in some health care centres. According to an online preprint article, the BCG vaccine could have the ability to prevent the infection with SARS CoV-2 [103]. In Japan, the BCG vaccination which was initiated in 1951, is very crucial for tuberculosis (TB) especially in areas with high or middle burden countries [104]. The Japanese Society for Vaccinology issued a notice that BCG vaccines for TB prevention among children may be considered as preference [99].

Due to lockdown in many cities and countries, the supply of a large number of anti-HIV drugs was depleted. So it is understandable that this would significantly affect the supply for the HIV infected patients [105]. The same aspect holds true for chloroquine, which is the first priority medication for systemic lupus erythematosus (SLE) also utilized for the treatment and prevention of malaria. According to some reports, chloroquine might be functional in case of COVID-19 [106]. In this manner, repurposing of drugs could deprive OI patients from their mandatory treatment.

Involuntary Risk Burden

In case of lack of proof or proven results, majorly considering DR with future planning may seem as a great strategy for communicable diseases. But such cases might manifold the risk probability without any proper control. Some well-known established theories in this respect are Consequentialism and utilitarianism. Treatments with respect to OI patients are prone to suffer in cases of sudden imbalance between demand and supplies for these drugs [99]. It is difficult to be justified only on the basis of consequentialism based on mortality rates among OI and NI patients. Moreover it is unjustified for OI patients to simply give their medical prescription only on the basis of this dilemma. It is akin to the plantation of other organs of a human body.

It is a known fact that transferring would reduce the chances of mortality when the whole population is considered, however with this, the chances of increased donors mortality rate will also rise. A study was done in England on public health where where asymptomatic patients were closely analysed and it was observed that patients with less immunity deviated from the trials and it was not ethically permissible [107, 108].

Regulatory Aspects and Ethical Issues in Drug Repurposing for COVID-19

When we consider COVID-19 pandemic, these regulatory aspects are defining factors for the application of these drugs. In case of any emergent needs, these drugs should be provided by these agencies without any delays and any kind of additional assessments for pros and cons [81]. Directive 2001/83/EC [109] gives a legal basis for drug repositioning based on EU directives. Three different actions that are carried out for the applications of repurposed drugs are centralised, decentralised and mutual recognition, out of which the centralised drugs are the most used [7, 110 - 114].

In the EU, there are two different pathways for repurposing; dossier pathway elaborated in article 8(3) of directive 2001/83/EC. It entails the administrative and other standard procedures and sequence of actions, including their bibliography. There is also a well-verified pathway for the applications under utilization from the last decade in the EU with well-defined acceptability and well-being [115]. In this option, applicants are not required to give clinical data in the dossier, and existing literature can be used. In these cases, 7-10 years are required for complete registration. Initially, more than one clinical trial is also needed for further registration [108, 115].

During emergency situations like the COVID-19 pandemic, all agencies must coordinate all registration and solutions for accelerated approvals. For countries like Japan, UK and US, it was seen that for early approvals, specific regulations were given without a visual clarification. In a similar case, remdesivir obtained Japan's authorisation under the Exceptional Approval Pathway [116, 117]. In the

US and the United Kingdom, its use was approved by another scheme known as Emergency Use authorisation [118]. The same pathway was used for conditional approval for remdesivir, and supplemental oxygen for pneumonia. In the latest report on COVID-19, it was clear that there was no effect on overall mortality, hospitalisation, *etc.*, by using remdesivir [111].

As a result, ethical issues are bound to arise in trials investigating repurposed drugs for the treatment and prevention of COVID-19, specifically when these agents are examined with less scientifically scientifically proven drugs. Many potential loose ends regarding both efficiency and security concerns may rise in this aspect when emergency sanctions of repositioned drugs are granted. The level of the pandemic and its social and health anomalies have shown the chance of a so-called tsunami of drug repurposing [119]. It was evident from the fact that around 550 drugs, from biological to oral medications, from supplements to herbal compositions, have been included in clinical trials due to the pandemic [7]. The point should be highlighted that most of these agents have well-proven indications, such as tocilizumab and hydroxychloroquine for rheumatoid arthritis or lopinavir/ritonavir for HIV [120].

Secondly, certain studies carried out at the beginning of the pandemic paved the basis for numerous drugs repurposed for COVID-19 [99]. Particularly, the topics entailed in the trials, including rushed approval of drugs, can be examples of actual requirements of investigated treatment. Moreover, if a repositioned drug cleared by the accelerated regulatory pathway proves to be the standard of care in the COVID-19 treatment, this could pave the way for the trial design of other drugs. As a result, experiments with large sample sizes and longer timelines will be needed to prove statistically dominant superiority or non-inferiority in comparison to the only supportive solutions to the disease. Another consideration is that endpoints might not always be taken by objective criteria for the accelerated approval pathway of the comparator [121]. Nevertheless, a large requirement for repositioned drugs showing less scope for any new indication may affect the distribution of supplies, depriving the public of an effective treatment. The risk of adverse outcomes should also be taken into account when repositioned agents without any clear efficacy are used for COVID-19 patients [122] (Fig. **2**).

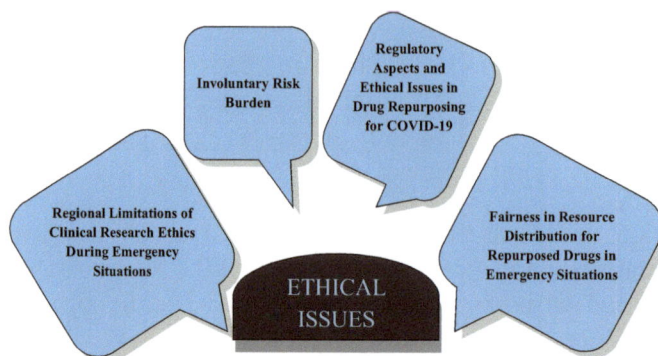

Fig. (2). This figure is demonstrating the ethical issues related to drug repurposing.

CONCLUSION

This chapter explored the repurposing of drugs and the challenges and ethical issues related to drug repurposing. Various narratives are available on drugs repurposed against the deadly COVID-19 and their contribution to clinical trials for the repurposing of drugs. The role of clinical trials has been significant in revealing the beneficial outcomes of Remdesivir, Tocilizumab, Dexamethasone, and Baricitinib. The deep search should be continued to explore the therapeutics for COVID-19 patients using potential anti-viral molecules, being evaluated in different phases of clinical trials. The purpose of drug repurposing has the ability to reduce the required time for a drug to reach the market, but it is still associated with scientific as well as regulatory challenges and careful ethical consideration.

CONSENT FOR PUBLICATION

Not applicable.

CONFLICT OF INTEREST

The author declares no conflict of interest, financial or otherwise.

ACKNOWLEDGEMENTS

Declared none.

REFERENCES

[1]   Tu YF, Chien CS, Yarmishyn AA, *et al.* A Review of SARS-CoV-2 and the Ongoing Clinical Trials. Int J Mol Sci 2020; 21(7): 2657.
[http://dx.doi.org/10.3390/ijms21072657] [PMID: 32290293]

[2]   Hossen MS, Barek MA, Jahan N, Safiqul Islam M. A Review on Current Repurposing Drugs for the Treatment of COVID-19: Reality and Challenges. SN Compr Clin Med 2020; 2(10): 1777-89.

[http://dx.doi.org/10.1007/s42399-020-00485-9] [PMID: 32904710]

[3]   Zhang Z, Zhou L, Xie N, *et al.* Overcoming cancer therapeutic bottleneck by drug repurposing. Signal Transduct Target Ther 2020; 5(1): 113.
[http://dx.doi.org/10.1038/s41392-020-00213-8] [PMID: 32616710]

[4]   Cui W, Yang K, Yang H. Recent Progress in the Drug Development Targeting SARS-CoV-2 Main Protease as Treatment for COVID-19. Front Mol Biosci 2020; 7: 616341.
[http://dx.doi.org/10.3389/fmolb.2020.616341] [PMID: 33344509]

[5]   Saul S, Einav S. Old Drugs for a New Virus: Repurposed Approaches for Combating COVID-19. ACS Infect Dis 2020; 6(9): 2304-18.
[http://dx.doi.org/10.1021/acsinfecdis.0c00343] [PMID: 32687696]

[6]   Singh TU, Parida S, Lingaraju MC, Kesavan M, Kumar D, Singh RK. Drug repurposing approach to fight COVID-19. Pharmacol Rep 2020; 72(6): 1479-508.
[http://dx.doi.org/10.1007/s43440-020-00155-6] [PMID: 32889701]

[7]   Sultana J, Crisafulli S, Gabbay F, Lynn E, Shakir S, Trifirò G. Challenges for Drug Repurposing in the COVID-19 Pandemic Era. Front Pharmacol 2020; 11: 588654.
[http://dx.doi.org/10.3389/fphar.2020.588654] [PMID: 33240091]

[8]   Wintergerst ES, Maggini S, Hornig DH. Immune-enhancing role of vitamin C and zinc and effect on clinical conditions. Ann Nutr Metab 2006; 50(2): 85-94.
[http://dx.doi.org/10.1159/000090495] [PMID: 16373990]

[9]   Prasad AS. Discovery of human zinc deficiency: its impact on human health and disease. Adv Nutr 2013; 4(2): 176-90.
[http://dx.doi.org/10.3945/an.112.003210] [PMID: 23493534]

[10]   Ho P, Zheng JQ, Wu CC, *et al.* Perspective Adjunctive Therapies for COVID-19: Beyond Antiviral Therapy. Int J Med Sci 2021; 18(2): 314-24.
[http://dx.doi.org/10.7150/ijms.51935] [PMID: 33390800]

[11]   Youssef DA, Miller CWT, El-Abbassi AM, *et al.* Antimicrobial implications of vitamin D. Dermatoendocrinol 2011; 3(4): 220-9.
[http://dx.doi.org/10.4161/derm.3.4.15027] [PMID: 22259647]

[12]   Ali N. Role of vitamin D in preventing of COVID-19 infection, progression and severity. J Infect Public Health 2020; 13(10): 1373-80.
[http://dx.doi.org/10.1016/j.jiph.2020.06.021] [PMID: 32605780]

[13]   Annweiler C, Beaudenon M, Gautier J, *et al.* COVIT-TRIAL study group. COvid-19 and high-dose VITamin D supplementation TRIAL in high-risk older patients (COVIT-TRIAL): study protocol for a randomized controlled trial. Trials 2020; 21(1): 1031.
[http://dx.doi.org/10.1186/s13063-020-04928-5] [PMID: 33371905]

[14]   Bae JH, Choe HJ, Holick MF, Lim S. Association of vitamin D status with COVID-19 and its severity. Rev Endocr Metab Disord 2022; 23(3): 579-99.
[http://dx.doi.org/10.1007/s11154-021-09705-6] [PMID: 34982377]

[15]   Prietl B, Treiber G, Pieber T, Amrein K. Vitamin D and immune function. Nutrients 2013; 5(7): 2502-21.
[http://dx.doi.org/10.3390/nu5072502] [PMID: 23857223]

[16]   Jolliffe DA, Camargo CA, Sluyter JD, *et al.* Vitamin D supplementation to prevent acute respiratory infections: systematic review and meta-analysis of aggregate data from randomised controlled trials 2020; 2020.07.14.20152728. Internet https://www.medrxiv.org/content/10.1101/2020.07.14.2015 2728v3
[http://dx.doi.org/10.1101/2020.07.14.20152728]

[17]   Prasad AS. Impact of the discovery of human zinc deficiency on health. J Am Coll Nutr 2009; 28(3): 257-65.

[http://dx.doi.org/10.1080/07315724.2009.10719780] [PMID: 20150599]

[18]   Valletta A, Iozia LM, Leonelli F. Impact of Environmental Factors on Stilbene Biosynthesis. Plants 2021; 10(1): 90.
[http://dx.doi.org/10.3390/plants10010090] [PMID: 33406721]

[19]   Shahidi F, Ambigaipalan P. Phenolics and polyphenolics in foods, beverages and spices: Antioxidant activity and health effects – A review. J Funct Foods 2015; 18: 820-97.
[http://dx.doi.org/10.1016/j.jff.2015.06.018]

[20]   Wahedi HM, Ahmad S, Abbasi SW. Stilbene-based natural compounds as promising drug candidates against COVID-19. J Biomol Struct Dyn 2020; 1-10.
[http://dx.doi.org/10.1080/07391102.2020.1762743] [PMID: 32345140]

[21]   Paciello F, Fetoni AR, Mezzogori D, *et al.* The dual role of curcumin and ferulic acid in counteracting chemoresistance and cisplatin-induced ototoxicity. Sci Rep 2020; 10(1): 1063.
[http://dx.doi.org/10.1038/s41598-020-57965-0] [PMID: 31974389]

[22]   Tahmasebi S, El-Esawi MA, Mahmoud ZH, *et al.* Immunomodulatory effects of nanocurcumin on Th17 cell responses in mild and severe COVID□19 patients. J Cell Physiol 2021; 236(7): 5325-38.
[http://dx.doi.org/10.1002/jcp.30233] [PMID: 33372280]

[23]   Wen CC, Kuo YH, Jan JT, *et al.* Specific plant terpenoids and lignoids possess potent antiviral activities against severe acute respiratory syndrome coronavirus. J Med Chem 2007; 50(17): 4087-95.
[http://dx.doi.org/10.1021/jm070295s] [PMID: 17663539]

[24]   Rattis BAC, Ramos SG, Celes MRN. Curcumin as a Potential Treatment for COVID-19. Front Pharmacol 2021; 12: 675287.
[http://dx.doi.org/10.3389/fphar.2021.675287] [PMID: 34025433]

[25]   Vallee BL, Falchuk KH. The biochemical basis of zinc physiology. Physiol Rev 1993; 73(1): 79-118.
[http://dx.doi.org/10.1152/physrev.1993.73.1.79] [PMID: 8419966]

[26]   Foster M, Samman S. Zinc and regulation of inflammatory cytokines: implications for cardiometabolic disease. Nutrients 2012; 4(7): 676-94.
[http://dx.doi.org/10.3390/nu4070676] [PMID: 22852057]

[27]   Wessels I, Rolles B, Rink L. The Potential Impact of Zinc Supplementation on COVID-19 Pathogenesis. Front Immunol 2020; 11: 1712.
[http://dx.doi.org/10.3389/fimmu.2020.01712] [PMID: 32754164]

[28]   Prasad AS. Zinc in human health: effect of zinc on immune cells. Mol Med 2008; 14(5-6): 353-7.
[http://dx.doi.org/10.2119/2008-00033.Prasad] [PMID: 18385818]

[29]   Prasad AS, Halsted JA, Nadimi M. Syndrome of iron deficiency anemia, hepatosplenomegaly, hypogonadism, dwarfism and geophagia. Am J Med 1961; 31(4): 532-46.
[http://dx.doi.org/10.1016/0002-9343(61)90137-1] [PMID: 14488490]

[30]   Todd WR, Elvehjem CA, Hart EB. Zinc in the nutrition of the rat. Am J Physiol 1933; 107(1): 146-56.
[http://dx.doi.org/10.1152/ajplegacy.1933.107.1.146]

[31]   Prasad AS. Zinc in human health: effect of zinc on immune cells. Mol Med 2008; 14(5-6): 353-7.
[http://dx.doi.org/10.2119/2008-00033.Prasad] [PMID: 18385818]

[32]   Prasad AS, Miale A Jr, Farid Z, Sandstead HH, Schulert AR. Zinc metabolism in patients with the syndrome of iron deficiency anemia, hepatosplenomegaly, dwarfism, and hypognadism. J Lab Clin Med 1963; 61: 537-49.
[PMID: 13985937]

[33]   Prasad AS, Meftah S, Abdallah J, *et al.* Serum thymulin in human zinc deficiency. J Clin Invest 1988; 82(4): 1202-10.
[http://dx.doi.org/10.1172/JCI113717] [PMID: 3262625]

[34]   Beck FWJ, Kaplan J, Fine N, Handschu W, Prasad AS. Decreased expression of CD73 (ecto-5-

-nucleotidase) in the CD8+ subset is associated with zinc deficiency in human patients. J Lab Clin Med 1997; 130(2): 147-56.
[http://dx.doi.org/10.1016/S0022-2143(97)90091-3] [PMID: 9280142]

[35] Beck FW, Prasad AS, Kaplan J, Fitzgerald JT, Brewer GJ. Changes in cytokine production and T cell subpopulations in experimentally induced zinc-deficient humans. Am J Physiol 1997; 272(6 Pt 1): E1002-7.
[PMID: 9227444]

[36] Arentz S, Hunter J, Yang G, *et al.* Zinc for the prevention and treatment of SARS-CoV-2 and other acute viral respiratory infections: a rapid review. Adv Integr Med 2020; 7(4): 252-60.
[http://dx.doi.org/10.1016/j.aimed.2020.07.009] [PMID: 32837895]

[37] Skalny A, Rink L, Ajsuvakova O, *et al.* Zinc and respiratory tract infections: Perspectives for COVID□19 (Review). Int J Mol Med 2020; 46(1): 17-26.
[http://dx.doi.org/10.3892/ijmm.2020.4575] [PMID: 32319538]

[38] te Velthuis AJW, van den Worm SHE, Sims AC, Baric RS, Snijder EJ, van Hemert MJ. Zn(2+) inhibits coronavirus and arterivirus RNA polymerase activity *in vitro* and zinc ionophores block the replication of these viruses in cell culture. PLoS Pathog 2010; 6(11): e1001176.
[http://dx.doi.org/10.1371/journal.ppat.1001176] [PMID: 21079686]

[39] Boron B, Hupert J, Barch DH, *et al.* Effect of zinc deficiency on hepatic enzymes regulating vitamin A status. J Nutr 1988; 118(8): 995-1001.
[http://dx.doi.org/10.1093/jn/118.8.995] [PMID: 3404291]

[40] Mammadova-Bach E, Braun A. Zinc Homeostasis in Platelet-Related Diseases. Int J Mol Sci 2019; 20(21): 5258.
[http://dx.doi.org/10.3390/ijms20215258] [PMID: 31652790]

[41] Vu T, Fredenburgh J, Weitz J. Zinc: An important cofactor in haemostasis and thrombosis. Thromb Haemost 2013; 109(3): 421-30.
[http://dx.doi.org/10.1160/TH12-07-0465] [PMID: 23306381]

[42] Zhang L, Liu Y. Potential interventions for novel coronavirus in China: A systematic review. J Med Virol 2020; 92(5): 479-90.
[http://dx.doi.org/10.1002/jmv.25707] [PMID: 32052466]

[43] Kumar A, Kubota Y, Chernov M, Kasuya H. Potential role of zinc supplementation in prophylaxis and treatment of COVID-19. Med Hypotheses 2020; 144: 109848.
[http://dx.doi.org/10.1016/j.mehy.2020.109848] [PMID: 32512490]

[44] Rosenkranz E, Metz CHD, Maywald M, *et al.* Zinc supplementation induces regulatory T cells by inhibition of Sirt-1 deacetylase in mixed lymphocyte cultures. Mol Nutr Food Res 2016; 60(3): 661-71.
[http://dx.doi.org/10.1002/mnfr.201500524] [PMID: 26614004]

[45] Lin F, Young HA. Interferons: Success in anti-viral immunotherapy. Cytokine Growth Factor Rev 2014; 25(4): 369-76.
[http://dx.doi.org/10.1016/j.cytogfr.2014.07.015] [PMID: 25156421]

[46] Ntyonga-Pono MP. COVID-19 infection and oxidative stress: an under-explored approach for prevention and treatment? Pan Afr Med J 2020; 35 (Suppl. 2): 12.
[http://dx.doi.org/10.11604/pamj.supp.2020.35.2.22877] [PMID: 32528623]

[47] Prasad AS, Bao B, Beck FWJ, Sarkar FH. Zinc-suppressed inflammatory cytokines by induction of A20-mediated inhibition of nuclear factor-κB. Nutrition 2011; 27(7-8): 816-23.
[http://dx.doi.org/10.1016/j.nut.2010.08.010] [PMID: 21035309]

[48] Wellinghausen N, Martin M, Rink L. Zinc inhibits interleukin-1-dependent T cell stimulation. Eur J Immunol 1997; 27(10): 2529-35.
[http://dx.doi.org/10.1002/eji.1830271010] [PMID: 9368606]

[49]   Samad N, Sodunke TE, Abubakar AR, *et al.* The Implications of Zinc Therapy in Combating the COVID-19 Global Pandemic. J Inflamm Res 2021; 14: 527-50.
[http://dx.doi.org/10.2147/JIR.S295377] [PMID: 33679136]

[50]   Blanco-Melo D, Nilsson-Payant BE, Liu W-C, *et al.* SARS-CoV-2 launches a unique transcriptional signature from *in vitro*, *ex vivo*, and *in vivo* systems 2020; 2020.03.24.004655. Internet https://www.biorxiv.org/content/10.1101/2020.03.24.004655v1
[http://dx.doi.org/10.1101/2020.03.24.004655]

[51]   Berg K, Bolt G, Andersen H, Owen TC. Zinc potentiates the antiviral action of human IFN-alpha tenfold. J Interferon Cytokine Res 2001; 21(7): 471-4.
[http://dx.doi.org/10.1089/10799900152434330] [PMID: 11506740]

[52]   Cakman I, Kirchner H, Rink L. Zinc supplementation reconstitutes the production of interferon-alpha by leukocytes from elderly persons. J Interferon Cytokine Res 1997; 17(8): 469-72.
[http://dx.doi.org/10.1089/jir.1997.17.469] [PMID: 9282827]

[53]   Ziegler CGK, Allon SJ, Nyquist SK, *et al.* SARS-CoV-2 Receptor ACE2 Is an Interferon-Stimulated Gene in Human Airway Epithelial Cells and Is Detected in Specific Cell Subsets across Tissues. Cell 2020; 181(5): 1016-1035.e19.
[http://dx.doi.org/10.1016/j.cell.2020.04.035] [PMID: 32413319]

[54]   Tan DX, Hardeland R. Targeting Host Defense System and Rescuing Compromised Mitochondria to Increase Tolerance against Pathogens by Melatonin May Impact Outcome of Deadly Virus Infection Pertinent to COVID-19. Molecules 2020; 25(19): 4410.
[http://dx.doi.org/10.3390/molecules25194410] [PMID: 32992875]

[55]   Salles C. Correspondence COVID-19: Melatonin as a potential adjuvant treatment. Life Sci 2020; 253: 117716.
[http://dx.doi.org/10.1016/j.lfs.2020.117716] [PMID: 32334009]

[56]   Anderson G, Maes M, Markus RP, Rodriguez M. Ebola virus: Melatonin as a readily available treatment option. J Med Virol 2015; 87(4): 537-43.
[http://dx.doi.org/10.1002/jmv.24130] [PMID: 25611054]

[57]   Shneider A, Kudriavtsev A, Vakhrusheva A. Can melatonin reduce the severity of COVID-19 pandemic? Int Rev Immunol 2020; 39(4): 153-62.
[http://dx.doi.org/10.1080/08830185.2020.1756284] [PMID: 32347747]

[58]   Reiter RJ, Tan DX, Fuentes-Broto L. Melatonin: a multitasking molecule. Prog Brain Res 2010; 181: 127-51.
[http://dx.doi.org/10.1016/S0079-6123(08)81008-4] [PMID: 20478436]

[59]   Crespo I, San-Miguel B, Sánchez DI, *et al.* Melatonin inhibits the sphingosine kinase 1/sphingosine---phosphate signaling pathway in rabbits with fulminant hepatitis of viral origin. J Pineal Res 2016; 61(2): 168-76.
[http://dx.doi.org/10.1111/jpi.12335] [PMID: 27101794]

[60]   Pierpaoli W, Yi C. The involvement of pineal gland and melatonin in immunity and aging I. Thymus-mediated, immunoreconstituting and antiviral activity of thyrotropin-releasing hormone. J Neuroimmunol 1990; 27(2-3): 99-109.
[http://dx.doi.org/10.1016/0165-5728(90)90059-V] [PMID: 2159021]

[61]   S M-L, N V, L C-B *et al.* High intensity light increases olfactory bulb melatonin in Venezuelan equine encephalitis virus infection. Neurochemical research [Internet]. 2001 Mar [cited 2021 Dec 20];26(3). Available from: https://pubmed.ncbi.nlm.nih.gov/11495546/

[62]   Cardinali DP. High doses of melatonin as a potential therapeutic tool for the neurologic sequels of covid-19 infection. Melatonin Research 2020; 3(3): 311-7.
[http://dx.doi.org/10.32794/mr11250064]

[63]   Cross KM, Landis DM, Sehgal L, Payne JD. Melatonin for the Early Treatment of COVID-19: A

Narrative Review of Current Evidence and Possible Efficacy. Endocr Pract 2021; 27(8): 850-5.
[http://dx.doi.org/10.1016/j.eprac.2021.06.001] [PMID: 34119679]

[64]   Campos LA, Cipolla-Neto J, Amaral FG, Michelini LC, Bader M, Baltatu OC. The Angiotensin-melatonin axis. Int J Hypertens 2013; 2013: 1-7.
[http://dx.doi.org/10.1155/2013/521783] [PMID: 23365722]

[65]   Ameri A, Asadi MF, Kamali M, *et al.* Evaluation of the effect of melatonin in patients with COVID-19-induced pneumonia admitted to the Intensive Care Unit: A structured summary of a study protocol for a randomized controlled trial. Trials 2021; 22(1): 194.
[http://dx.doi.org/10.1186/s13063-021-05162-3] [PMID: 33685474]

[66]   Rodríguez-Rubio M, Figueira JC, Acuña-Castroviejo D, Borobia AM, Escames G, de la Oliva P. A phase II, single-center, double-blind, randomized placebo-controlled trial to explore the efficacy and safety of intravenous melatonin in patients with COVID-19 admitted to the intensive care unit (MelCOVID study): a structured summary of a study protocol for a randomized controlled trial. Trials 2020; 21(1): 699.
[http://dx.doi.org/10.1186/s13063-020-04632-4] [PMID: 32758298]

[67]   Dose-Ranging Study to Assess the Safety and Efficacy of Melatonin in Outpatients Infected With COVID-19.
https://clinicaltrials.gov/show/NCT047847542021.
https://www.cochranelibrary.com/central/doi/10.1002/central/CN-02236879/full

[68]   Safety and Efficacy of Melatonin in Outpatients Infected With COVID-19.
https://clinicaltrials.gov/show/NCT044744832020.
https://www.cochranelibrary.com/central/doi/10.1002/central/CN-02137224/related-content

[69]   Baghdasht MSB. 2020.https://clinicaltrials.gov/ct2/show/NCT04409522

[70]   Efficacy of Melatonin in the Prophylaxis of Coronavirus Disease.
2019.https://clinicaltrials.gov/show/NCT04353128
https://www.cochranelibrary.com/central/doi/10.1002/central/CN-02103276/full

[71]   Lancaster General Hospital. 2020.https://clinicaltrials.gov/ct2/show/NCT04530539

[72]   Piovezan RD. Adjuvant Therapeutic Effects of Melatonin Agonist on Hospitalized Patients With Confirmed or Suspected COVID-19 [Internet]. clinicaltrials.gov; 2020 Jul [cited 2021 Dec 16]. Report No.: NCT04470297. Available from: https://clinicaltrials.gov/ct2/show/NCT04470297

[73]   Liu W, Zhang S, Nekhai S, Liu S. Depriving Iron Supply to the Virus Represents a Promising Adjuvant Therapeutic Against Viral Survival. Curr Clin Microbiol Rep 2020; 7(2): 13-9.
[http://dx.doi.org/10.1007/s40588-020-00140-w] [PMID: 32318324]

[74]   Polamreddy P, Gattu N. The drug repurposing landscape from 2012 to 2017: evolution, challenges, and possible solutions. Drug Discov Today 2019; 24(3): 789-95.
[http://dx.doi.org/10.1016/j.drudis.2018.11.022] [PMID: 30513339]

[75]   Darrow JJ, Avorn J, Kesselheim AS. FDA Approval and Regulation of Pharmaceuticals, 1983-2018. JAMA 2020; 323(2): 164-76.
[http://dx.doi.org/10.1001/jama.2019.20288] [PMID: 31935033]

[76]   Oprea TI, Mestres J. Drug repurposing: far beyond new targets for old drugs. AAPS J 2012; 14(4): 759-63.
[http://dx.doi.org/10.1208/s12248-012-9390-1] [PMID: 22826034]

[77]   Wittich CM, Burkle CM, Lanier WL. Ten common questions (and their answers) about off-label drug use. Mayo Clin Proc 2012; 87(10): 982-90.
[http://dx.doi.org/10.1016/j.mayocp.2012.04.017] [PMID: 22877654]

[78]   Bhattacharya S, Saha CN. Intellectual property rights: An overview and implications in pharmaceutical industry. J Adv Pharm Technol Res 2011; 2(2): 88-93.
[http://dx.doi.org/10.4103/2231-4040.82952] [PMID: 22171299]

[79] Drug Repurposing and the COVID-19 Pandemic [Internet]. [cited 2021 Dec 16]. Available from: https://www.wipo.int/wipo_magazine/en/2020/02/article_0004.html

[80] Verbaanderd C, Rooman I, Meheus L, Huys I. On-Label or Off-Label? Overcoming Regulatory and Financial Barriers to Bring Repurposed Medicines to Cancer Patients. Front Pharmacol 2020; 10: 1664.
[http://dx.doi.org/10.3389/fphar.2019.01664] [PMID: 32076405]

[81] Pushpakom S, Iorio F, Eyers PA, *et al.* Drug repurposing: progress, challenges and recommendations. Nat Rev Drug Discov 2019; 18(1): 41-58.
[http://dx.doi.org/10.1038/nrd.2018.168] [PMID: 30310233]

[82] Facilitating adoption of off-patent, repurposed medicines into NHS clinical practice [Internet]. Association of Medical Research Charities. [cited 2021 Dec 16]. Available from: https://www.amrc.org.uk/blog/facilitating-adoption-of-off-patent-repur-osed-medicines-into-nhs-clinical-practice

[83] Repurposing drugs: the opportunity and the challenges [Internet]. Association of Medical Research Charities. [cited 2021 Dec 16]. Available from: https://www.amrc.org.uk/blog/repurposing-drugs-t-e-opportunity-and-the-challenges

[84] Allarakhia M. Open-source approaches for the repurposing of existing or failed candidate drugs: learning from and applying the lessons across diseases. Drug Des Devel Ther 2013; 7: 753-66.
[http://dx.doi.org/10.2147/DDDT.S46289] [PMID: 23966771]

[85] Ritchie MD, Holzinger ER, Li R, Pendergrass SA, Kim D. Methods of integrating data to uncover genotype–phenotype interactions. Nat Rev Genet 2015; 16(2): 85-97.
[http://dx.doi.org/10.1038/nrg3868] [PMID: 25582081]

[86] Talevi A, Bellera CL. Challenges and opportunities with drug repurposing: finding strategies to find alternative uses of therapeutics. Expert Opin Drug Discov 2020; 15(4): 397-401.
[http://dx.doi.org/10.1080/17460441.2020.1704729] [PMID: 31847616]

[87] Engel JC, Ang KKH, Chen S, Arkin MR, McKerrow JH, Doyle PS. Image-based high-throughput drug screening targeting the intracellular stage of Trypanosoma cruzi, the agent of Chagas' disease. Antimicrob Agents Chemother 2010; 54(8): 3326-34.
[http://dx.doi.org/10.1128/AAC.01777-09] [PMID: 20547819]

[88] Planer JD, Hulverson MA, Arif JA, Ranade RM, Don R, Buckner FS. Synergy testing of FDA-approved drugs identifies potent drug combinations against Trypanosoma cruzi. PLoS Negl Trop Dis 2014; 8(7): e2977.
[http://dx.doi.org/10.1371/journal.pntd.0002977] [PMID: 25033456]

[89] Sykes ML, Avery VM. Development and application of a sensitive, phenotypic, high-throughput image-based assay to identify compound activity against Trypanosoma cruzi amastigotes. Int J Parasitol Drugs Drug Resist 2015; 5(3): 215-28.
[http://dx.doi.org/10.1016/j.ijpddr.2015.10.001] [PMID: 27120069]

[90] Hammond DJ, Cover B, Gutteridge WE. A novel series of chemical structures active *in vitro* against the trypomastigote form of Trypanosoma cruzi. Trans R Soc Trop Med Hyg 1984; 78(1): 91-5.
[http://dx.doi.org/10.1016/0035-9203(84)90184-6] [PMID: 6369655]

[91] Hammond DJ, Hogg J, Gutteridge WE. Trypanosoma cruzi: Possible control of parasite transmission by blood transfusion using amphiphilic cationic drugs. Exp Parasitol 1985; 60(1): 32-42.
[http://dx.doi.org/10.1016/S0014-4894(85)80020-5] [PMID: 3926530]

[92] Alirol E, Schrumpf D, Amici Heradi J, *et al.* Nifurtimox-eflornithine combination therapy for second-stage gambiense human African trypanosomiasis: Médecins Sans Frontières experience in the Democratic Republic of the Congo. Clin Infect Dis 2013; 56(2): 195-203.
[http://dx.doi.org/10.1093/cid/cis886] [PMID: 23074318]

[93] Hunter AJ, Lee WH, Bountra C. Open innovation in neuroscience research and drug discovery. Brain

Neurosci Adv 2018; 2.
[http://dx.doi.org/10.1177/2398212818799270] [PMID: 32166150]

[94] Oprea TI, Bauman JE, Bologa CG, *et al.* Drug repurposing from an academic perspective. Drug Discov Today Ther Strateg 2011; 8(3-4): 61-9.
[http://dx.doi.org/10.1016/j.ddstr.2011.10.002] [PMID: 22368688]

[95] Parvathaneni V, Gupta V. Utilizing drug repurposing against COVID-19 – Efficacy, limitations, and challenges. Life Sci 2020; 259: 118275.
[http://dx.doi.org/10.1016/j.lfs.2020.118275] [PMID: 32818545]

[96] Breckenridge A, Jacob R. Overcoming the legal and regulatory barriers to drug repurposing. Nat Rev Drug Discov 2019; 18(1): 1-2.
[http://dx.doi.org/10.1038/nrd.2018.92] [PMID: 29880920]

[97] Emanuel EJ, Wendler D, Grady C. What makes clinical research ethical? JAMA 2000; 283(20): 2701-11.
[http://dx.doi.org/10.1001/jama.283.20.2701] [PMID: 10819955]

[98] Bierer BE, White SA, Barnes JM, Gelinas L. Ethical Challenges in Clinical Research During the COVID-19 Pandemic. J Bioeth Inq 2020; 17(4): 717-22.
[http://dx.doi.org/10.1007/s11673-020-10045-4] [PMID: 33169251]

[99] Ino H, Nakazawa E, Akabayashi A. Drug Repurposing for COVID-19: Ethical Considerations and Roadmaps. Camb Q Healthc Ethics 2021; 30(1): 51-8.
[http://dx.doi.org/10.1017/S0963180120000481] [PMID: 32498751]

[100] Emanuel EJ, Persad G, Upshur R, *et al.* Fair Allocation of Scarce Medical Resources in the Time of Covid-19. N Engl J Med 2020; 382(21): 2049-55.
[http://dx.doi.org/10.1056/NEJMsb2005114] [PMID: 32202722]

[101] Iwabuchi K, Yoshie K, Kurakami Y, Takahashi K, Kato Y, Morishima T. Therapeutic potential of ciclesonide inhalation for COVID-19 pneumonia: Report of three cases. J Infect Chemother 2020; 26(6): 625-32.
[http://dx.doi.org/10.1016/j.jiac.2020.04.007] [PMID: 32362440]

[102] Matsuyama S, Kawase M, Nao N, *et al.* The Inhaled Steroid Ciclesonide Blocks SARS-CoV-2 RNA Replication by Targeting the Viral Replication-Transcription Complex in Cultured Cells. J Virol 2020; 95(1): e01648-20.
[http://dx.doi.org/10.1128/JVI.01648-20] [PMID: 33055254]

[103] Can a century-old TB vaccine steel the immune system against the new coronavirus? [Internet]. [cited 2021 Dec 16]. Available from: https://www.science.org/content/article/can-century-old-tb-vac-ine-steel-immune-system-against-new-coronavirus

[104] Yamamoto S, Yamamoto T. Historical review of BCG vaccine in Japan. Jpn J Infect Dis 2007; 60(6): 331-6.
[PMID: 18032829]

[105] World Health Organization. Combined global demand forecasts for antiretroviral medicines and HIV diagnostics in low- and middle-income countries from 2015 to 2020 [Internet]. World Health Organization; 2016 [cited 2021 Dec 16]. 66 p. Available from: https://apps.who.int/iris/handle/10665/250088

[106] Wang M, Cao R, Zhang L, *et al.* Remdesivir and chloroquine effectively inhibit the recently emerged novel coronavirus (2019-nCoV) *in vitro.* Cell Res 2020; 30(3): 269-71.
[http://dx.doi.org/10.1038/s41422-020-0282-0] [PMID: 32020029]

[107] COVID-19: investigation and initial clinical management of possible cases [Internet]. GOV.UK. [cited 2021 Dec 21]. Available from: https://www.gov.uk/government/publications/wuhan-nove--coronavirus-initial-investigation-of-possible-cases/investigation-and-initial-clinical-ma-agement-of-possible-cases-of-wuhan-novel-coronavirus-wn-cov-infection

[108] China Clinical Trial Registry-World Health Organization International Clinical Trial Registration Platform Class I Registration Body [Internet]. [cited 2021 Dec 21]. Available from: http://www.chictr.org.cn/showproj.aspx?proj=48684

[109] Bayoumy AB, de Boer NKH, Ansari AR, Crouwel F, Mulder CJJ. Unrealized potential of drug repositioning in Europe during COVID-19 and beyond: a physician's perspective. J Pharm Policy Pract 2020; 13(1): 45.
[http://dx.doi.org/10.1186/s40545-020-00249-9] [PMID: 32695427]

[110] Omolo CA, Soni N, Fasiku VO, Mackraj I, Govender T. Update on therapeutic approaches and emerging therapies for SARS-CoV-2 virus. Eur J Pharmacol 2020; 883: 173348.
[http://dx.doi.org/10.1016/j.ejphar.2020.173348] [PMID: 32634438]

[111] Mohanty S, Harun AI Rashid M, Mridul M, Mohanty C, Swayamsiddha S, Swayamsiddha S. Application of Artificial Intelligence in COVID-19 drug repurposing. Diabetes Metab Syndr 2020; 14(5): 1027-31.
[http://dx.doi.org/10.1016/j.dsx.2020.06.068] [PMID: 32634717]

[112] Mangione W, Falls Z, Melendy T, Chopra G, Samudrala R. Shotgun drug repurposing biotechnology to tackle epidemics and pandemics. Drug Discov Today 2020; 25(7): 1126-8.
[http://dx.doi.org/10.1016/j.drudis.2020.05.002] [PMID: 32405249]

[113] Ke YY, Peng TT, Yeh TK, *et al.* Artificial intelligence approach fighting COVID-19 with repurposing drugs. Biomed J 2020; 43(4): 355-62.
[http://dx.doi.org/10.1016/j.bj.2020.05.001] [PMID: 32426387]

[114] Richardson P, Griffin I, Tucker C, *et al.* Baricitinib as potential treatment for 2019-nCoV acute respiratory disease. Lancet 2020; 395(10223): e30-1.
[http://dx.doi.org/10.1016/S0140-6736(20)30304-4] [PMID: 32032529]

[115] Research C for DE and. Product Development Under the Animal Rule [Internet]. U.S. Food and Drug Administration. FDA; 2020 [cited 2021 Dec 16]. Available from: https://www.fda.gov/regulatory-information/search-fda-guidance-documents/product-development-under-animal-rule

[116] Beigel JH, Tomashek KM, Dodd LE, Mehta AK, Zingman BS, Kalil AC, *et al.* 2020. Remdesivir for the Treatment of Covid-19 — Final Report. New England Journal of Medicine [Internet]. 2020 May 22 [cited 2021 Dec 22]; Available from: https://www.nejm.org/doi/10.1056/NEJMoa2007764

[117] Saint-Raymond A, Sato J, Kishioka Y, Teixeira T, Hasslboeck C, Kweder SL. Remdesivir emergency approvals: a comparison of the U.S., Japanese, and EU systems. Expert Rev Clin Pharmacol 2020; 13(10): 1095-101.
[http://dx.doi.org/10.1080/17512433.2020.1821650] [PMID: 32909843]

[118] Research C for DE and. FDA's approval of Veklury (remdesivir) for the treatment of COVID-19—the science of safety and effectiveness. FDA [Internet]. 2021 Sep 30 [cited 2021 Dec 16]; Available from: https://www.fda.gov/drugs/news-events-human-drugs/fdas-approval-veklury-remdesivir-tr-atment-covid-19-science-safety-and-effectiveness

[119] Mucke HAM. COVID-19 and the Drug Repurposing Tsunami. Assay Drug Dev Technol 2020; 18(5): 211-4.
[http://dx.doi.org/10.1089/adt.2020.996] [PMID: 32551883]

[120] Scuccimarri R, Sutton E, Fitzcharles MA. Hydroxychloroquine: A Potential Ethical Dilemma for Rheumatologists during the COVID-19 Pandemic. J Rheumatol 2020; 47(6): 783-6.
[http://dx.doi.org/10.3899/jrheum.200369] [PMID: 32241801]

[121] Singh JA, Upshur REG. The granting of emergency use designation to COVID-19 candidate vaccines: implications for COVID-19 vaccine trials. Lancet Infect Dis 2021; 21(4): e103-9.
[http://dx.doi.org/10.1016/S1473-3099(20)30923-3] [PMID: 33306980]

[122] Gatti M, De Ponti F. Drug Repurposing in the COVID-19 Era: Insights from Case Studies Showing Pharmaceutical Peculiarities. Pharmaceutics 2021; 13(3): 302.

CHAPTER 3

Repurposed Drugs Against SARS-CoV-2 Replication in COVID-19

Kavita Verma[1], Yoganchal Mishra[1], Sarika Singh[2], Neha Kapoor[3] and Neelam Yadav[1,*]

[1] *Department of Biochemistry, Dr. Rammanohar Lohia Avadh University, Ayodhya-224001, India*

[2] *Neurosciences an Ageing Biology and Toxicology and Experimental Medicine Division, CSIR-Central Drug Research Institute, Lucknow-226031, India*

[3] *Department of Chemistry, Hindu College, University of Delhi-110007, India*

Abstract: COVID-19 caused by severe acute respiratory syndrome coronavirus 2(SARS-CoV -2), has emerged as a global health problem. It was first reported in Wuhan city of China, in December 2019. Unfortunately, no specific and effective drug is available to treat SARS-CoV-2 infection in patients. There is an urgent need to control COVID-19pandemic. Research & development of novel molecules is a time-consuming and labour-intensive procedure in the midst of a pandemic. The aim of drug repurposing is to find a therapeutically effective molecule from a library of pre-existing compounds. In the present article, a large number of anti-viral drugs with their potential efficacy in inhibiting replication of virus by targeting the virus S protein (Spike protein), 3-chymotrypsin-like protease (3CLpro), RNA-dependent RNA polymerase (RdRp) and papain-like protease (PLpro), which play an important role in the replication cycle and pathogenesis of coronaviruses, were assessed as possible treatment options against SARS-CoV-2 infected COVID-19 patients. The continuing SARS-CoV-2 epidemic emphasises the importance of efficient anti-viral medications that can be administered swiftly to decrease morbidity, death, and viral transmission. Several breakthroughs in the development of COVID-19 treatment options might be made by repurposing widely active anti-viral medicines and chemicals that are known to suppress viral replication of related viruses.

Keywords: Anti-viral drugs, COVID-19, Drug repurposing, Remdesivir, Replication, SARS-CoV-2.

INTRODUCTION

COVID-19, a novel coronavirus illness, has become a pandemic danger to human health. It is a respiratory illness that causes dry cough, lethargy, fever, muscular

* **Corresponding author Neelam Yadav:** Department of Biochemistry, Dr. Rammanohar Lohia Avadh University, Ayodhya-224001, Tel: +91 9453731722, India; E-mail:neelam2k4@gmail.com

Tabish Qidwai (Ed.)

pains, and shortness of breath, as well as pneumonia in certain cases [1, 2]. It can induce acute respiratory distress syndrome, which is a severe inflammation of the lung in which fluid builds up within and around the lungs, causing septic trauma owing to a significant drop in blood pressure and the body's parts being underfed for oxygen. This corona virus has an incubation period of 1 to 14 days. The degree of symptoms varies from patient to patient. Due to weakened or damaged immune systems, the elderly, children under the age of six, and individuals with a medical history of asthma, diabetes, or heart disease are especially sensitive to this condition. In December 2019, Wuhan, Hubei Province, China, was the centre of the epidemic [2, 3]. WHO declared this outbreak a Public Health Emergency of International Concern on January 30, 2020, because of its rapid spread and estimated reproductive number (Ro) of 2.2. As of March 20, 2020, it had reached approximately 187 countries (2, 66,073 confirmed cases) and 11,184 confirmed fatalities with a 4.4 ofcase fatality rate (CFT) [4].

Severe acute respiratory syndrome coronavirus 2 (SARS-CoV-2) is the virus that causes COVID-19. Middle East respiratory sickness (MERS) virus (MERS-CoV) and SARS-CoV are two more related agents [5, 6]. They infiltrate the pulmonary epithelial cells, deliver their nucleocapsid, and hijack the cellular machinery to multiply in the cytoplasm, attacking the patient's lower respiratory system. The heart, kidneys, liver, gastrointestinal tract, and central nervous system are all affected by the virus family. The Coronaviridae family of enveloped single-stranded, positive-strand ribonucleic acids includes SARS-CoV-2 (RNA) structure.

It is critical to find efficient medicinal chemicals in order to respond quickly to this pandemic viral illness. Presently, due to the urgent need to stop COVID-19 infection, therapeutic approaches for this pandemic include repurposing existing anti-viral drugs that have an effect on the replication of novel SARS-CoV -2 coronavirus [7]. Therapeutic methods for COVID-19 infection patients are divided into two groups based on their targets: (1) medications that target the SARS-CoV-2 life cycle and (2) therapies that have efficacy on the host cells or human immune system. In this chapter, we discuss repurposed drugs with anti-viral effects against SARS-CoV-2 replication, as these substances provide great efficacy for early treatment of COVID-19 by inhibiting the virus life cycle. In addition, it may work as suitable preventive measure, as reported for neuraminidase inhibitors in the influenza virus.

Currently, several clinical trials are ongoing in which many immunomodulators and anti-viral drugs are being investigated for the treatment of COVID-19 patients. These trials aim to decrease the morbidity and mortality rate of this infectious disease until an effective vaccine or drug is developed.

SARS-CoV-2 Genome Structure

The SARS-CoV -2 genome is made up of a single-stranded positive-sense RNA [8]. The SARS-CoV -2 genome was recently sequenced and published to the NCBI genome database (NC 045512.2) with a size of 29.9 kb [9]. SARS-CoV-2 has 13-15 open reading frames (ORFs) with a total of 30,000 nucleotides in its genetic composition. The genome has a GC content of 38 percent and 11 protein-coding genes along with 12 expressed proteins. The genomic organisation of ORFs is strikingly similar to that of SARS-CoV and MERS-CoV [10, 11]. The ORFs are classified as replicase and protease (1a -1b), as well as important S, E, M, and N proteins, in a 5 ′ - 3 ′ order of occurrence and are regarded major drug/vaccine targets. These gene products play critical roles in the viral entrance, fusion, and host cell survival [12]. The SARS -CoV -2 genome is organised in a linear topology, with roughly 89 percent sequence similarity with other CoVs. The translated sequences of SARS-CoV -2 proteins were found in GenBank (Accession ID: NC 045512.2)]. SARS-whole CoV-2's genome encodes a 7096-residue-long polyprotein that contains a variety of structural and non-structural proteins (NSPs). The viral genome's nucleotide content is mostly carried by two non-structural proteins (ORF1a and ORF1ab) and structural proteins. ORFs 1a and 1b encode polyproteins pp1a and pp1ab, respectively, with polyprotein pp1ab encoded *via* the ribosomal frameshift mechanism of gene 1b. These polyproteins are processed by proteinases (virally encoded), which result in the production of 16 proteins that are highly conserved across all CoVs in the same family.

SARS-CoV-2 Infection and Pathogenesis

In COVID-19 infection, SARS-CoV-2 infects its host cells by identifying the angiotensin-converting enzyme 2 (ACE2) enzymes [9]. ACE2 is a transmembrane protein found in the cells of the lungs, arteries, veins, intestines, heart and kidneys [13]. ACE2 operates as a vasodepressor in the pulmonary epithelium, stabilizing the effect of its homologous enzyme ACE1, which behaves as a vasoconstrictor, and both enzymes make up the oxygen-sensitive renin-angiotensin-system (RAS) [14]. The dynamic equilibrium between the expression of ACE1 and ACE2 regulates the RAS system in normoxia. However, in human pulmonary artery smooth muscle cells (hPASMC), ACE1 is upregulated by the hypoxia-inducible factor 1 (HIF-1) (a master regulator of the response to hypoxia) during chronic hypoxia (oxygen 2 percent for 12 days), but ACE2 expression is significantly reduced [15]. Similar results were found in male rats exposed to altitudes of 4,500 metres, which revealed higher levels of ACE1 and reduced expression of ACE2 in cardiac cells after 28 days [16]. As the level of expression of ACE2 (in pulmonary epithelial cells) has been shown to be certainly correlated with the rate of SARS-CoVinfection [9, 17 - 19], these findings are extremely important for the pathogenesis of COVID-19. These findings strongly imply that people who live at high altitudes (*i.e.*, continuously exhibiting hypoxic stages) have lower amounts of ACE2 in their lungs (and other organs). As a result, successful acclimatisation to the environment(high-altitude) may make regional residents less vulnerable to SARS-CoV-2 viral infection and protect them from developing the illness that defines acute respiratory distress syndrome.

SARS-CoV-2 Genome Replication and Transcription

SARS-CoV-2 infection begins with virion attachment to target cells, which is mediated mostly by interactions of thelarge surface glycoproteins(S proteins) with the host-cell-surface receptors called angiotensin-converting enzyme2(ACE2) [20 - 23]. The S protein undergoes proteolytic cleavage by transmembrane protease serine 2 (TMPRSS2), which causes structural changes in the S protein, leads to the fusing of the viral and host membranes and the release of viral gRNA into the cytoplasm (Fig. **1**). Both ACE2 and TMPRSS2 are expressed in a variety of cell types, with a high level of expression in epithelial and endothelial cells in the lungs and gut, allowing SARSCoV-2 to infect a variety of important organs. SARS-CoV-2 is an RNA virus that replicates only in the cytoplasm of infected cells, where cellular proteases unzip the viral genome from bound viral N proteins. The viral +gRNA then functions as an mRNA for ORF1a and ORF1b translation, as well as a template RNA for RNA transcription. Following interactions between the nsps, which include viral RNA-dependent RNA polymerase(RdRP), which is derived from cleaved ORF1a and ORF1b polyproteins, a replication and transcription complex (RTC) is formed on the template +gRNA for virus gRNA transcription and single guide RNA(sgRNA) synthesis inside virus infection-induced double-membrane vesicles (DMVs) [24, 25]. The viral structural and auxiliary proteins are encoded by the freshly synthesised sgRNAs released by the DMV. Finally, freshly generated gRNA is encapsidated with N proteins, wrapped in a viral envelope and discharged from infected cells [26].

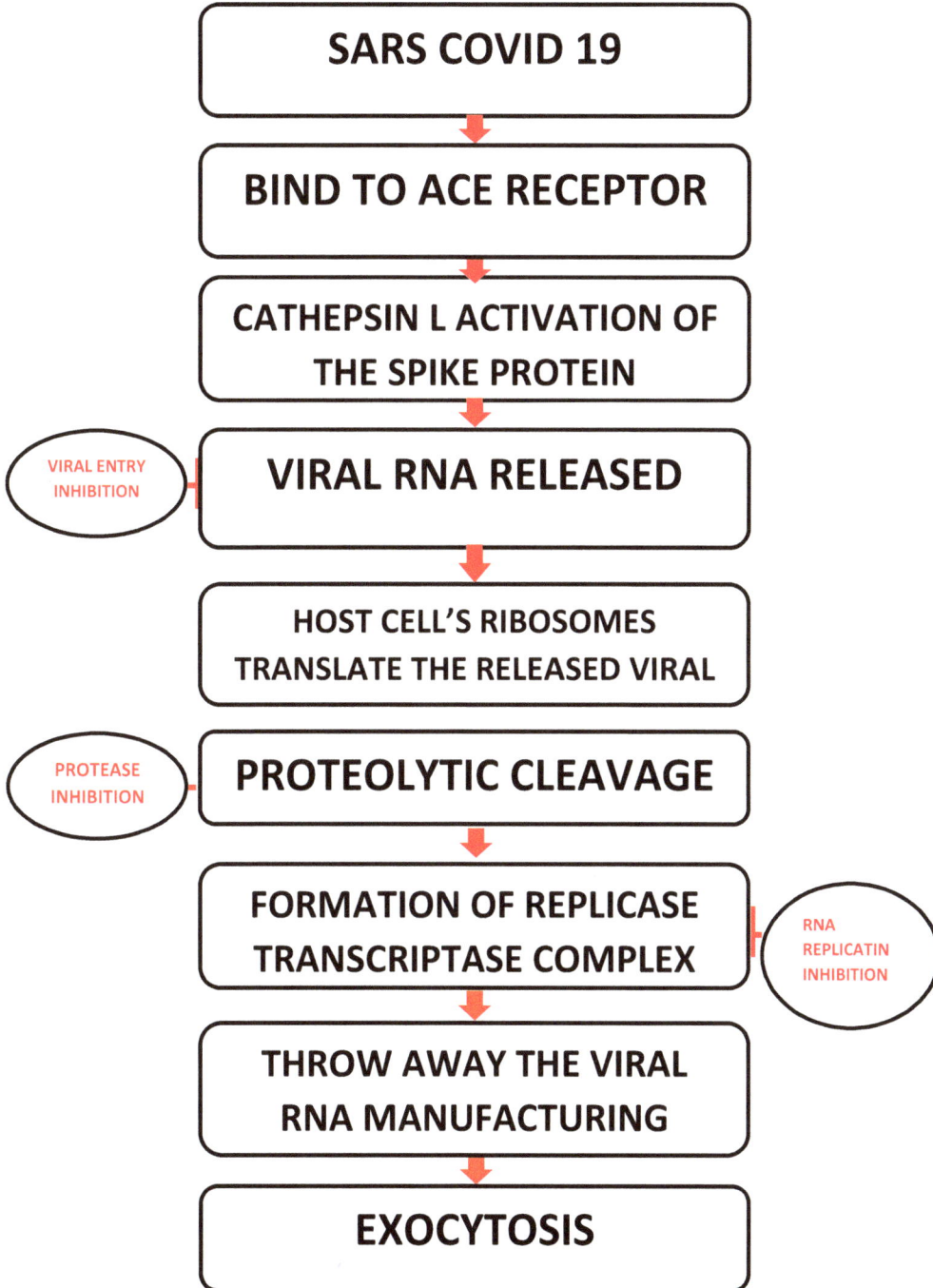

Fig. (1). SARS-CoV-2 replication cycle and anti-viral medication targets.

The viral spike protein binds to the ACE2 receptor, which allows SARS-CoV-2 to attach to its host cell. The exposed S2 subunit initiates fusion of the viral and host cell membranes after proteolytic cleavage of the S1 domain by the membrane-anchored serine protease TMPRSS2. SARS-CoV-2 can also infect the host cell after endosomal absorption and cathepsin L activation of the spike protein. The host cell's ribosomes translate the released viral RNA. The primary protease of the virus cleaves the polyproteins pp1a/pp1ab (3C-like proteinase). The replicase–transcriptase complex, which is formed by released non-structural proteins, kicks off the viral RNA manufacturing machinery. Exocytosis releases new particles made up of viral structural proteins and genomic RNA. The replication cycle of SARS-CoV-19 occurs by inhibition of [1, 2] Viral Entry [3], Protease Inhibition and [4] RNA Replication Inhibition.

Repurposed Drugs Against SARS-CoV-2 Replication

Repurposed drugs with anti-SARS-CoV2 activity can be classified into one of four categories based on their mode of action: 1)- substances that prevent viral entry into host cells, 2)- inhibitors of viral proteases, 3)- inhibitors of viral replicase, 4)- other compounds elicit multiple effects, or its specific mechanism of action in SARS-CoV-2 is unknown (Table **1**).

Prevention of SARS-CoV-2 Entry into the Host Cell

The spike (S) protein is divided into functional S1 and S2 fragments by furin-like protease (host cell-derived protease). The S2 subunit initiates viral entry, which needs S protein priming by proteolytic cleavage of the S1 subunit. The serine protease TMPRSS2 and the endosomal cysteine proteases cathepsin B and L are required for viral entry in cell lines, as shown in other coronaviruses [27, 28].

Several studies, however, suggest that TMPRSS2 preferentially drives cell entrance *via* the cell surface or early endosomes, and that TMPRSS2's proteolytic cleavage of the S-protein is required for host infection [29, 30]. As a result, blocking TMPRSS2 and/or cathepsin B and L appears to be a good target for preventing viral entrance.

Nafamostat/Camostat

TMPRSS2 is a cell membrane-anchored serine protease from the type II transmembrane serine protease family. The catalytic mechanism of these proteases is based on a trio of three amino acids (serine, aspartate, and histidine) found in highly conserved sequence patterns [31]. Serine proteases are tightly controlled by endogenous inhibitors (such as a1/a2-antitrypsin and antithrombin III) and require the previous activation to achieve hemostasis under healthy settings. As a result, an imbalance can lead to a variety of pathological events, including thrombosis [32]. TMPRSS2's particular physiological roles, however, remain uncertain. Synthetic protease inhibitors, such as nafamostatmesilateor camostatmesilate, have been clinically tested in patients with pancreatitis (acute or chronic), which is pathophysiologically linked to abnormal activation of digestive enzymes inside the pancreas, including the trypsin (serine protease) [33, 34]. Serine protease inhibitors have been explored for their anti-viral effects on SARS-CoV-2 and other coronaviruses due to their ability to inhibit TMPRSS2. Camostat inhibited the entrance of vesicular stomatitis virus (VSV) pseudotyped particles (pseudovirions) containing the SARS-CoV-2 spike protein into the Caco-2 human epithelial colorectal adenocarcinoma cell line, human airway epithelial cells (HAE) and VeroTMPRSS2+ cells. Only when camostat was administered in conjunction with E-64d (a cathepsin B/L inhibitor), 100% viral entrance suppression was achieved, suggesting that SARS-CoV-2 can enter the host cell *via* both routes [28]. However, TMPRSS2 is required for viral pathogenesis and transmission while CatB/L activity is not; therefore, TMPRSS2 inhibition shows a sensible anti-viral tactic (Table **1**).

Table 1. Repurposed anti-viral drugs against SARS-CoV-2 replication in COVID-19.

Anti-viral Targets	Investigational Repurposed Drug	Primary Use	Active Against	Mechanism	Year of Discovery and Reference
Viral entry	Nafamostat	acute pancreatitis	MERS and SARS-CoV-2 replication cycle inhibition	Inhibits TMPRSS2 (host cells protease) and membrane fusion of virus	[77]
-	Umifenovir (Arbidol)	Influenza	Influenza	Inhibits membrane fusion	[40, 41]
-	Griffithsin	HIV	anti-viral (Broad-spectrum) effective against SARS MERS and HIV	Attached with glycoprotein present on surface of virus and inhibits viral entry (*e.g.*, SARS-CoV-2 S protein and HIV gp120)	[71]
-	Disulfiram	Chronic alcoholism	inhibition activity for MERS and SARS-CoV-2 and for HIV treatment	Inhibit the cleavage of viral polyprotein	[72]

(Table 1) cont.....

Anti-viral Targets	Investigational Repurposed Drug	Primary Use	Active Against	Mechanism	Year of Discovery and Reference
Viral protease	Lopinavir/ ritonavir	HIV treatment drug	Inhibit the life cycle of the SARS, MERS and SARS-CoV-2	Inhibiting replication of virus by high (binding) affinity to the viral protease	[63]
-	Nelfinavir	Approved Drug for HIV-1	Inhibition of replication cycle of SARS and SARS CoV-2	Effective inhibitor for viral protease (*e.g.* 3CLpro)	[73]
-	Danoprevir	Use to treat noncirrhotic genotype 1b HCV	Potential efficacy against SARS-CoV-2	Inhibits viral protease (*e.g.* 3CLpro)	[74]
RNA synthesis	Favipiravir (Avigan)	A guanine analog drug use to treat flu	Therapeutic efficacy against yellow fever virus, SARS-CoV-2 and influenza virus	viral RNA-dependent RNA polymerase (RdRp) inhibition	[62]
-	Ribavirin	Effective drug for RSV and HCV	Effective agaist SARS-CoV-2 and MERS	Inhibits the viral RNA synthesis (by viral mRNA capping) termination (*via* viral RdRp targeting)	[62]
-	Remdesivir	Drug (adenosine analog) for Ebola virus	Therapeutic efficacy against Ebola virus, Respiratory syncytial virus and other ss RNA viruses including MERS, RSV, SARS and SARS-CoV-2	Acts as a terminator of RNA-chain (after binding with viral RdRp)	[62]
-	Penciclovir	Effective drug for cold sores treatment caused by virus (herpes simplex)	Antibacterials antifungals and anti-virals	docked the protein (nsp12), which reigns the RNA-dependent RNA polymerase (action of SARS-CoV-2)	[62]

(Table 1) cont.....

Anti-viral Targets	Investigational Repurposed Drug	Primary Use	Active Against	Mechanism	Year of Discovery and Reference
-	Galidesivir	Drug (adenosine Analog) for HCV	Anti-viral action against many RNA viruses (*e.g.*, MER CoV, SARS-Co, Marburg and Ebola)	Inhibits the viral RNA polymerase and helps in transcription	[75]
Miscellaneous	Nitazoxanide	A drug for diarrhea	Broad-spectrum anti-viral	Pyruvate:ferredoxin oxidoreductase (PFOR) enzyme	[40]
-	Emetine	**A drug for amebiasis**	Antiparasitic drug	Inhibits both ribosomal and mitochondrial protein synthesis	[63]
-	Homoharringtonine	**Chronic myelogenous leukemia**	Cancer	Inhibits cell proliferation, migration and invasion, and promotes apoptosis in CRC by inactivating PI3K/AKT/mTOR signaling pathway.	[63]
-	Hydroxychloroquine	A drug used to treat discoid lupus erythematosus (DLE) or systemic lupus erythematosus (SLE or lupus)	Anti-malarial and anti-inflammatory actions	Affects the life cycle of the virus at the stage of cell entry and after-entry.	[76]
-	Cyclosporine A	Immunosuppressant	Immune-mediated diseases	Inhibits nuclear factor of activated T cells (NFAT) activity	[64]
-	Chloroquine	A drug to treat Malaria	Malaria	CQ affects the viral life cycle both at cell entry and post-entry stages.	[62]

(Table 1) cont.....

Anti-viral Targets	Investigational Repurposed Drug	Primary Use	Active Against	Mechanism	Year of Discovery and Reference
-	Berberine	A drug for diabetes	anti-inflammatory, anticancer, bacteriostatic, antioxidant, lipid-lowering and hypoglycemic effects	Inhibit DNA synthesis by affecting the activity of DNA topoisomerase	[64]

Nafamostat is a drug used for the treatment of acute pancreatitis. This drug has shown an anti-viral effect on MERS-CoV by regulating the host protease (TMPRSS2), essential for priming S protein and virus entry to the host cells [35]. A new finding demonstrates that nafamostat is very effective in inhibiting the fusion of the membrane of SARS-CoV-2 to the host cells. It might be a good therapeutic approach for COVID-19-infected patients [36].

Umifenovir

Umifenovir(a broad-spectrum anti-viral drug) has been licensed for the prevention and treatment of human influenza A and B infections in China and Russia [37]. Its anti-viral effect is hypothesised to be linked to a virus-mediated membrane fusion defect, which is required for viral entrance. Umifenovir appears to affect the negatively charged phospholipids in the host cell membrane, changing its physicochemical characteristics [38]. Furthermore, umifenovir has been found to interact with influenza virus hemagglutinin (HA) by blocking the pH-induced transition of HA into its functional form [39]. The efficacy of six presently available and approved anti-influenza medications (umifenovir, zanamivir, oseltamivir, laninamivir, peramivir, and baloxavir) against SARS-CoV-2 in Vero E6 cells was recently examined in the research. Only umifenovir(with an EC50 of 4.11 lM) effectively reduced SARS-CoV-2 replication among the medicines tested [40]. Another, *in vitro* investigation with an EC50 of 3.5 lM might replicate these findings [41]. Although, umifenovir showed anti-SARSCoV-2 efficacy *in vitro*, its therapeutic function in COVID-19 is unknown, and qualitative clinical trial outcomes are few. Retrospective evaluations show that there is now no discernible influence on clinical outcomes [42].

Anti-viral Approach by Targeting the SARS-CoV-2 Protease

The proteolytic cleavage of polyproteins and release of functional polypeptides by viral proteases is a critical step in SARS-CoV-2 replication. The replicase–transcriptase complex, which begins the viral RNA manufacturing machinery, is formed as a result of the released non-structural proteins. New infectious virus particles are produced from replicated genomic RNA and translated viral structural proteins, which are discharged from the infected host cell. The major protease (Mpro), also called 3C-like protease (3CLpro), cleaves the polyprotein (between Leu-Gln and Ser-Ala-Gly) in coronaviruses. This enzyme is an excellent anti-viral target as it is required for the replication of the virus [43, 44]. The toxicity of certain inhibitors is predicted to be restricted due to their inherent proteolytic activity and the lack of similar enzymes in humans. The combination of lopinavir and ritonavir has been the centre of attention among known protease inhibitors that have been repurposed for SARS-CoV-2, while other protease inhibitors (*e.g.*, darunavir) have shown little *in vitro* action at applicable dosages [45].

Lopinavir/Ritonavir

Lopinavir is a well-known anti-viral drug. Infections with the human immunodeficiency virus type 1(HIV-1) are treated with a combination of lopinavir and ritonavir (Kaletra). Both lopinavir and ritonavir are inhibitors of HIV-1 protease enzyme that use bond hydrolysis to break the HIV polyproteins Gag and Gag-Pol. Because ritonavir inhibits cytochrome P450-3A4 (CYP3A4), an enzyme that typically metabolises protease inhibitors, it is used to increase lopinavir's bioavailability [46]. SARS-CoV, MERS-CoV and human coronavirus 229E have all been tested *in vitro* with lopinavir [47].

Inhibition of Viral RNA Replicase

The replicase–transcriptase complex, which catalyses the production of viral RNA, may be produced after the proteolytic division of the polyproteins. The RdRp binds to the 3' end of the RNA strand and starts the synthesis process. In the elongation phase, the complementary RNA strand is created by repeating nucleotidyl transfer events. Several medicines have the ability to disrupt the RNA production process. The majority of the nucleoside/nucleotide analogues drugs have been repurposed and evaluated against SARS-CoV-2infection. During the elongation phase, these medicines compete with endogenous nucleosides and disrupt the replication of the virus. Following their insertion, nucleoside analogues cause a chain termination and a halt to RNA synthesis, which is required for the production of new viral particles.

Remdesivir

Remdesivir (GS-5734), amonophosphoramidate nucleoside prodrug, is originated to penetrate through the cell membrane and release its metabolite quickly [48]. Due to its capacity to circumvent an inefficient and rate-limiting initial phosphorylation step, remdesivir monophosphate (RDV-MP) is rapidly transformed into its active triphosphate form once it enters target cells [49]. The physiologically active remdesivir triphosphate (RDV-TP) serves as a substrate for the viral replicase (RdRp) in RNA viruses, where it competes with endogenous adenosine-triphosphate (ATP) for incorporation into elongating RNA strands. RDV-TP inhibits synthesis by inducing delayed chain termination, as reported for the Ebola virus (EBOV) [50], MERS-CoV [51], SARS-CoV, and SARS-CoV-2 [52]. When RDV-TP is incorporated into SARS-CoV-2, RNA production is stopped after three more nucleoside/nucleotide sites downstream [52]. Although, other analogues related to RDV have been under pharmacological modification and investigation for several years [53, 54]. The present drug for the management of viral diseases was first reported (2016) on the basis of the fatal EVD macaque model and preclinical data of cell-based assays [55].

Favipiravir

Favipiravir (T-705) is a derivative of pyrazine. It suppresses the RdRpof many RNA viruses. In the case of influenza, it was discovered that the active triphosphate form acts as a nucleotide analogue that competes with ATP and GTP for incorporation into the nascent RNA strand resulting in chain termination [56]. Favipiravir-TP acts as a competitive inhibitor of viral RdRp and also causes random point mutations, which eventually lead to deadly mutagenesis of the virus [57, 58]. Under *in vitro* condition, this drug has significant anti-viral activity against influenza A and B, and it is now licensed drug for the treatment of influenza infections in Japan [59, 60]. In addition, it showed wide anti-viral activity against many RNA viruses, including human metapneumovirus, respiratory syncytial virus, measles virus, human parainfluenza virus, and paramyxoviruses [61]. However, cell-based experiments checked effectiveness against SARS-CoV-2 and revealed minimal activity at high (micromolar) concentrations or no activity at the highest concentration [62 - 64].

Ribavirin

Ribavirin is a guanosine analogue that resembles favipiravir in structure. It inhibits viral RNA production by incorporating it into nascent RNA strands, just as other nucleoside or nucleotide analogues. However, other additional mechanisms may play a role in its anti-viral action. It has been demonstrated that ribavirin shows a mutagenic impact on the viral genome and reduces cellular GTP pools by interfering with cellular inosinmonophosphatde hydrogenase in the case of influenza [65, 66]. Ribavirin is an anti-viral medicine that is licensed for the management of chronic hepatitis C virus (HCV) infections in conjunction with other anti-viral treatments. Ribavirin has wide efficacy against RNA viruses, particularly those belonging to the flavivirus family [67]. Although, virtual molecular docking studies reveal that SARS-CoV-2 RdRp interacts with it, but it's effectiveness against SARS-CoV-2 is limited [64, 65]. This isn't unexpected as ribavirin has no anti-viral effect on related coronaviruses [68]. Therefore, ribavirin was not tested in humans.

Penciclovir

Penciclovir is also a guanosine analogue that has been licensed as a topical anti-viral drug for the management of viral infections(herpes simplex). It has a low bioavailability. Famciclovir(prodrug version of pencivlovir) has improved bioavailability and is effective against herpes infections, such as herpes zoster. According to a test based on virtual binding in the nsp12 homology model, Pencivlovir attaches to SARS-CoV-2 RdRp with high affinity than RDV [69]. Despite this, it has modest effectiveness against SARS-CoV-2 (EC50 96 M)under *in vitro* conditions [60]. In addition, there have been no more preclinical or clinical investigations with penciclovir or its prodrug famciclovir for COVID-19 therapy.

CONCLUSION

SARS-CoV-2 has created a global outbreak of novel, extremely contagious COVID-19. It has become a serious health concern for the general public. However, information about SARS-CoV-2 and its sickness is still restricted. This infection necessitates immediate research and development of novel anti-viral medicines. There is currently no specific medicine that can be used to treat this illness. As developing a new medication takes time, repurposing broad-spectrum anti-viral medicines might be a good way to treat quickly. It is difficult to find specific and efficient drugs to respond quickly to this viral illness pandemic. Therapeutic approaches for the treatment of COVID-19 patients are divided into two categories based on their targets: 1) drugs that target the SARS-CoV-2 replication cycle and 2) therapies that have efficacy on the human immune system and host cells. This chapter discusses repurposed drugs with anti-viral efficacy against SARS-CoV-2 infection. In addition, these compounds provide great potential for the early management of COVID-19 by inhibiting viral replication and may even be suitable for preventive approaches. Many compounds were examined *in vitro* for their capacity to minimise cytopathologic effects on Vero E6 cells or their direct anti-viral effects on SARS-CoV-2 replication. However, only thirteen of them have shown any activity against SARS-CoV-2 so far. To date, none of the repurposed entry and viral protease inhibitors has demonstrated persuasive data to support clinical development as a single treatment against COVID-19. Other nucleotide or nucleoside analogues (that target the viral RdRp), such as penciclovir, favipiravir or ribavirin, were evaluated but found less effective against SARS-CoV-2 infection. Viral protease inhibitors were also checked, but only lopinavir exhibited any activity against the virus. Recent *in vitro* investigations have shown that drugs, including nitazoxanide, cyclosporine A, emetine, and homoharringtonine, which have distinct and largely unknown mechanisms of anti-viral activity, have substantial anti-SARSCoV-2 characteristics. However, none of these drugs have been thoroughly tested in animal models or clinical studies. As a result, remdesivir is the only anti-viral medicine that has been shown to be effective in both preclinical and clinical trials. In the latter case, it shortens the time it takes to recuperate and may minimise mortality.

FUTURE PERSPECTIVE

Regrettably, there is no particular effective therapy for SARS-CoV-2 infection in COVID-19 patients at this time. Due to the quick spread of SARS-CoV-2 and the high fatality rate of this unique pandemic illness, it is critical to manage this highly infectious disease by discovering new therapies or utilising anti-viral that have the capacity to block virus replication. Several clinical trials are underway throughout the world to develop effective treatment drugs to combat this unique virus by inhibiting the viral replication cycle by targeting structural and/or non-structural proteins. Extracellular vesicles (EVs) as a potential drug-delivery method were reported for repurposing anti-virals drugs against SARS-CoV-2 replication in COVID-19 patients [70]. EVs are excellent transporters of biological molecules, including DNA, RNA, miRNA, and other tiny molecules.This research reveals that anti-viral medicines encapsulated in EVs as natural nanocarriers can target particular tissues, increasing their effectiveness and safety in COVID-19 patients [70]. The future aims to finish clinical trials and determine the effective, cost-efficient, tolerable and safe, anti-viral medicines and/or vaccines for the treatment of Covid- 19 pandemic.

CONSENT FOR PUBLICATION

Not applicable.

CONFLICT OF INTEREST

The author declares no conflict of interest, financial or otherwise.

ACKNOWLEDGEMENTS

Declared none.

REFERENCES

[1]   Rothan HA, Byrareddy SN. The epidemiology and pathogenesis of coronavirus disease (COVID-19) outbreak. J Autoimmun 2020; 109: 102433.
[http://dx.doi.org/10.1016/j.jaut.2020.102433]

[2]   Liu C, Zhou Q, Li Y, *et al.* Research and Development on therapeutic agents and vaccines for COVID-19 and related human coronavirus diseases. ACS Cent Sci 2020; 6(3): 315-31.
[http://dx.doi.org/10.1021/acscentsci.0c00272] [PMID: 32226821]

[3]   Bogoch A, Watts A, Thomas-Bachli C, *et al.* Pneumonia of unknown etiology in Wuhan, China: potential for international spread *via* commercial air travel. J Travel Med 2020;27(2):taaa008.
[http://dx.doi.org/10.1093/jtm/taaa008]

[4]   Organization WH. Coronavirus Disease (COVID-2019) Situation Reports-61, 21 March 2020.

[5]   Elfiky AA. Anti-HCV, nucleotide inhibitors, repurposing against COVID-19. Life Sci 2020; 248: 117477.
[http://dx.doi.org/10.1016/j.lfs.2020.117477] [PMID: 32119961]

[6]   Wrapp D, NianShuang W, Kizzmekia SC, *et al.* Cryo-EM structure of the 2019- nCoV spike in the prefusion conformation. Science 2020;367(6483):1260-1263.
[http://dx.doi.org/10.1126/ science.abb2507]

[7]   Mitj'a O andClotet B. Use of anti-viral drugs to reduce COVID-19 transmission. Lancet Glob Health 2020; 8(5): e639-40.
[http://dx.doi.org/10.1016/S2214-109X(20)30114-5] [PMID: 32199468]

[8]   Wu F, Zhao S, Yu B, *et al.* A new coronavirus associated with human respiratory disease in China. Nature 2020; 579(7798): 265-9.
[http://dx.doi.org/10.1038/s41586-020-2008-3] [PMID: 32015508]

[9]   Lu R, Zhao X, Li J, *et al.* Genomic characterisation and epidemiology of 2019 novel coronavirus: implications for virus origins and receptor binding. Lancet 2020; 395(10224): 565-74.
[http://dx.doi.org/10.1016/S0140-6736(20)30251-8] [PMID: 32007145]

[10]   Lu R, Wang Y, Wang W, *et al.* Complete genome sequence of Middle East respiratory syndrome coronavirus (MERS -CoV) from the first imported MERS -CoV case in China. Genome Announc 2015; 3: e00818-00815.

[11]   Rota PA, Oberste MS, Monroe SS, *et al.* Characterization of a novel coronavirus associated with severe acute respiratory syndrome. Science 2003; 300(5624): 1394-9.
[http://dx.doi.org/10.1126/science.1085952] [PMID: 12730500]

[12]   Tong TR. Drug targets in severe acute respiratory syndrome (SARS) virus and other coronavirus infections, Infectious Disorders -Drug Targets (Formerly Current Drug Targets-Infectious Disorders) 2009; 9: 223-45.

[13]   Hamming I, Timens W, Bulthuis MLC, Lely AT, Navis GJ, van Goor H. Tissue distribution of ACE2 protein, the functional receptor for SARS coronavirus. A first step in understanding SARS pathogenesis. J Pathol 2004; 203(2): 631-7.
[http://dx.doi.org/10.1002/path.1570] [PMID: 15141377]

[14]   Hampl V, Herget J, Bíbová J, *et al.* Intrapulmonary activation of the angiotensin-converting enzyme type 2/angiotensin 1-7/G-protein-coupled Mas receptor axis attenuates pulmonary hypertension in Ren-2 transgenic rats exposed to chronic hypoxia. Physiol Res 2015; 64(1): 25-38.
[http://dx.doi.org/10.33549/physiolres.932861] [PMID: 25194138]

[15]   Zhang R, Wu Y, Zhao M, *et al.* Role of HIF-1α in the regulation ACE and ACE2 expression in hypoxic human pulmonary artery smooth muscle cells. Am J Physiol Lung Cell Mol Physiol 2009; 297(4): L631-40.
[http://dx.doi.org/10.1152/ajplung.90415.2008] [PMID: 19592460]

[16]   Dang Z, Su S, Jin G, *et al*. TsantanSumtang attenuated chronic hypoxia-induced right ventricular structure remodeling and fibrosis by equilibrating local ACE-AngII-AT1R/ACE2-Ang1-7-Mas axis in rat. J Ethnopharmacol 250; 112470.
[http://dx.doi.org/10.1016/j.jep.2019.112470]

[17]   Jia HP, Look DC, Shi L, *et al*. ACE2 receptor expression and severe acute respiratory syndrome coronavirus infection depend on differentiation of human airway epithelia. J Virol2005; 79 (23): 14614–21.
[http://dx.doi.org/10.1128/JVI.79. 23.14614-14621]

[18]   Ren LL, Wang YM, Wu ZQ, *et al*. Identification of a novel coronavirus causing severe pneumonia in human: a descriptive study. Chin Med J (Engl) 2020;133(9):1015-1024.
[http://dx.doi.org/10.1097/CM9.0000000000000722]

[19]   Rothan HA andByrareddy SN. The epidemiology and pathogenesis of coronavirus disease (COVID-19) outbreak. J Autoimmun 2020; 102433.
[http://dx.doi.org/10.1016/j.jaut.2020.102433]

[20]   Zhou P, Yang XL, Wang XG, *et al*. A pneumonia outbreak associated with a new coronavirus of probable bat origin. Nature 2020; 579(7798): 270-3.
[http://dx.doi.org/10.1038/s41586-020-2012-7] [PMID: 32015507]

[21]   Wrapp D, Wang N, Corbett KS, *et al*. Cryo-EM structure of the 2019-nCoV spike in the prefusion conformation. Science 2020; 367(6483): 1260-3.
[http://dx.doi.org/10.1126/science.abb2507] [PMID: 32075877]

[22]   Walls AC, Park YJ, Tortorici MA, Wall A, McGuire AT, Veesler D. Structure, function, and antigenicity of the SARS-CoV-2 spike glycoprotein. Cell 2020; 181(2): 281-292.e6.
[http://dx.doi.org/10.1016/j.cell.2020.02.058] [PMID: 32155444]

[23]   Yan R, Zhang Y, Li Y, Xia L, Guo Y, Zhou Q. Structural basis for the recognition of SARS-CoV-2 by full-length human ACE2. Science 2020; 367(6485): 1444-8.
[http://dx.doi.org/10.1126/science.abb2762] [PMID: 32132184]

[24]   Wolff G, Melia CE, Snijder EJ, Bárcena M. Double-membrane vesicles as platforms for viral replication. Trends Microbiol 2020; 28(12): 1022-33.
[http://dx.doi.org/10.1016/j.tim.2020.05.009] [PMID: 32536523]

[25]   Klein S, Cortese M, Winter SL, *et al*. SARS-CoV-2 structure and replication characterized by *in situ* cryo-electron tomography. Nat Commun 2020; 11(1): 5885.
[http://dx.doi.org/10.1038/s41467-020-19619-7] [PMID: 33208793]

[26]   Hartenian E, Nandakumar D, Lari A, Ly M, Tucker JM, Glaunsinger BA. The molecular virology of coronaviruses. J Biol Chem 2020; 295(37): 12910-34.
[http://dx.doi.org/10.1074/jbc.REV120.013930] [PMID: 32661197]

[27]   Kawase M, Shirato K, van der Hoek L, Taguchi F, Matsuyama S. Simultaneous treatment of human bronchial epithelial cells with serine and cysteine protease inhibitors prevents severe acute respiratory syndrome coronavirus entry. J Virol 2012; 86(12): 6537-45.
[http://dx.doi.org/10.1128/JVI.00094-12] [PMID: 22496216]

[28]   Hoffmann M, Kleine-Weber H, Schroeder S, *et al*. SARS-CoV-2 cell entry depends on ACE2 and TMPRSS2 and is blocked by a clinically proven protease inhibitor. Cell 2020; 181(2): 271-280.e8. a
[http://dx.doi.org/10.1016/j.cell.2020.02.052] [PMID: 32142651]

[29]   Shirato K, Kawase M, Matsuyama S. Wild-type human coronaviruses prefer cell-surface TMPRSS2 to endosomal cathepsins for cell entry. Virology 2018; 517: 9-15.
[http://dx.doi.org/10.1016/j.virol.2017.11.012] [PMID: 29217279]

[30]   Iwata-Yoshikawa N, Okamura T, Shimizu Y, Hasegawa H, Takeda M, Nagata N. TMPRSS2 contributes to virus spread and immunopathology in the airways of murine models after coronavirus infection. J Virol 2019; 93(6): e01815-18.

[http://dx.doi.org/10.1128/JVI.01815-18] [PMID: 30626688]

[31]   Antalis TM, Bugge TH, Wu Q. Membrane-anchored serine proteases in health and disease. Prog Mol Biol Transl Sci 2011; 99: 1-50.
[http://dx.doi.org/10.1016/D978-0-12-385504-6.00001-4] [PMID: 21238933]

[32]   Rau JC, Beaulieu LM, Huntington JA, Church FC. Serpins in thrombosis, hemostasis and fibrinolysis. J Thromb Haemost 2007; 5 (Suppl. 1): 102-15.
[http://dx.doi.org/10.1111/j.1538-7836.2007.02516.x] [PMID: 17635716]

[33]   Chang JH, Lee IS, Kim HK, *et al*. Nafamostat for Prophylaxis against Post-Endoscopic Retrograde Cholangiopancreatography Pancreatitis Compared with Gabexate. Gut Liver 2009; 3(3): 205-10.
[http://dx.doi.org/10.5009/gnl.2009.3.3.205] [PMID: 20431747]

[34]   Ramsey ML, Nuttall J, Hart PA. A phase 1/2 trial to evaluate the pharmacokinetics, safety, and efficacy of NI-03 in patients with chronic pancreatitis: study protocol for a randomized controlled trial on the assessment of camostat treatment in chronic pancreatitis (TACTIC). Trials 2019; 20(1): 501.
[http://dx.doi.org/10.1186/s13063-019-3606-y] [PMID: 31412955]

[35]   Yamamoto M, Matsuyama S, Li X, *et al*. Identification of nafamostat as a potent inhibitor of Middle East respiratory syndromecoronavirus S protein-mediated membrane fusion using the split-protei--based cell-cell fusion assay. Antimicrob Agents Chemother 2016; 60(11): 6532-9.
[http://dx.doi.org/10.1128/AAC.01043-16] [PMID: 27550352]

[36]   Balfour H. Nafamostat inhibits SARS-CoV-2 infection, preventing COVID-19 transmission. Drug Target Review. NEWS 2020. http://www.drugtargetreview.com/news/58915/

[37]   Boriskin Y, Leneva I, Pécheur EI, Polyak S. Arbidol: a broad-spectrum antiviral compound that blocks viral fusion. Curr Med Chem 2008; 15(10): 997-1005.
[http://dx.doi.org/10.2174/092986708784049658] [PMID: 18393857]

[38]   Villalaín J. Membranotropic effects of arbidol, a broad anti-viral molecule, on phospholipid model membranes. J Phys Chem B 2010; 114(25): 8544-54.
[http://dx.doi.org/10.1021/jp102619w] [PMID: 20527735]

[39]   Leneva IA, Russell RJ, Boriskin YS, Hay AJ. Characteristics of arbidol-resistant mutants of influenza virus: Implications for the mechanism of anti-influenza action of arbidol. Antiviral Res 2009; 81(2): 132-40.
[http://dx.doi.org/10.1016/j.antiviral.2008.10.009] [PMID: 19028526]

[40]   Wang X, Cao R, Zhang H, *et al*. The anti-influenza virus drug, arbidol is an efficient inhibitor of SARS-CoV-2 *in vitro*. Cell Discov 2020; 6(1): 28. b
[http://dx.doi.org/10.1038/s41421-020-0169-8] [PMID: 32373347]

[41]   Pizzorno A, Padey B, Dubois J, *et al*. *In vitro* evaluation of antiviral activity of single and combined repurposable drugs against SARS-CoV-2. Antiviral Res 2020; 181: 104878.
[http://dx.doi.org/10.1016/j.antiviral.2020.104878] [PMID: 32679055]

[42]   Huang D, Yu H, Wang T, Yang H, Yao R, Liang Z. Efficacy and safety of umifenovir for coronavirus disease 2019 (COVID-19): A systematic review and meta-analysis. J Med Virol 2020; 192: E734-44.
[PMID: 32617989]

[43]   Anand K, Ziebuhr J, Wadhwani P, Mesters JR, Hilgenfeld R. Coronavirus main proteinase (3CLpro) structure: basis for design of anti-SARS drugs. Science 2003; 300(5626): 1763-7.
[http://dx.doi.org/10.1126/science.1085658] [PMID: 12746549]

[44]   Zhang L, Lin D, Sun X, *et al*. Crystal structure of SARS-CoV-2 main protease provides a basis for design of improved α-ketoamide inhibitors. Science 2020; 368(6489): 409-12. b
[http://dx.doi.org/10.1126/science.abb3405] [PMID: 32198291]

[45]   De Meyer S, Bojkova D, Cinatl J, *et al*. Lack of antiviral activity of darunavir against SARS-CoV-2. Int J Infect Dis 2020; 97: 7-10.
[http://dx.doi.org/10.1016/j.ijid.2020.05.085] [PMID: 32479865]

[46]   Sham HL, Kempf DJ, Molla A, *et al.* ABT-378, a highly potent inhibitor of the human immunodeficiency virus protease. Antimicrob Agents Chemother 1998; 42(12): 3218-24.
[http://dx.doi.org/10.1128/AAC.42.12.3218] [PMID: 9835517]

[47]   de Wilde AH, Jochmans D, Posthuma CC, *et al.* Screening of an FDA-approved compound library identifies four small-molecule inhibitors of Middle East respiratory syndrome coronavirus replication in cell culture. Antimicrob Agents Chemother 2014; 58(8): 4875-84.
[http://dx.doi.org/10.1128/AAC.03011-14] [PMID: 24841269]

[48]   Jordheim LP, Durantel D, Zoulim F, Dumontet C. Advances in the development of nucleoside and nucleotide analogues for cancer and viral diseases. Nat Rev Drug Discov 2013; 12(6): 447-64.
[http://dx.doi.org/10.1038/nrd4010] [PMID: 23722347]

[49]   Murakami E, Niu C, Bao H, *et al.* The mechanism of action of beta-D-2′-deoxy-2′-fluo-o-2′-C-methylcytidine involves a second metabolic pathway leading to beta-D-2′-deoxy-2′-flu-ro-2′-C-methyluridine 5′-triphosphate, a potent inhibitor of the hepatitis C virus RNA-dependent RNA polymerase. Antimicrob Agents Chemother 2008; 52(2): 458-64.
[http://dx.doi.org/10.1128/AAC.01184-07] [PMID: 17999967]

[50]   Tchesnokov E, Feng J, Porter D, Götte M. Mechanism of inhibition of ebola virus RNA-dependent RNA Polymerase by Remdesivir. Viruses 2019; 11(4): 326.
[http://dx.doi.org/10.3390/v11040326] [PMID: 30987343]

[51]   Gordon CJ, Tchesnokov EP, Feng JY, Porter DP, Götte M. The antiviral compound remdesivir potently inhibits RNA-dependent RNA polymerase from Middle East respiratory syndrome coronavirus. J Biol Chem 2020; 295(15): 4773-9. a
[http://dx.doi.org/10.1074/jbc.AC120.013056] [PMID: 32094225]

[52]   Gordon CJ, Tchesnokov EP, Woolner E, *et al.* Remdesivir is a direct-acting antiviral that inhibits RNA-dependent RNA polymerase from severe acute respiratory syndrome coronavirus 2 with high potency. J Biol Chem 2020; 295(20): 6785-97. b
[http://dx.doi.org/10.1074/jbc.RA120.013679] [PMID: 32284326]

[53]   Cho A, Saunders OL, Butler T, *et al.* Synthesis and antiviral activity of a series of 1′-substituted 4-az--7,9-dideazaadenosine C-nucleosides. Bioorg Med Chem Lett 2012; 22(8): 2705-7.
[http://dx.doi.org/10.1016/j.bmcl.2012.02.105] [PMID: 22446091]

[54]   Seley-Radtke KL, Yates MK. The evolution of nucleoside analogue antivirals: A review for chemists and non-chemists. Part 1: Early structural modifications to the nucleoside scaffold. Antiviral Res 2018; 154: 66-86.
[http://dx.doi.org/10.1016/j.antiviral.2018.04.004] [PMID: 29649496]

[55]   Warren TK, Jordan R, Lo MK, *et al.* Therapeutic efficacy of the small molecule GS-5734 against Ebola virus in rhesus monkeys. Nature 2016; 531(7594): 381-5.
[http://dx.doi.org/10.1038/nature17180] [PMID: 26934220]

[56]   Sangawa H, Komeno T, Nishikawa H, *et al.* Mechanism of action of T-705 ribosyl triphosphate against influenza virus RNA polymerase. Antimicrob Agents Chemother 2013; 57(11): 5202-8.
[http://dx.doi.org/10.1128/AAC.00649-13] [PMID: 23917318]

[57]   Vanderlinden E, Vrancken B, Van Houdt J, *et al.* Distinct effects of T-705 (Favipiravir) and ribavirin on influenza virus replication and viral RNA synthesis. Antimicrob Agents Chemother 2016; 60(11): 6679-91.
[http://dx.doi.org/10.1128/AAC.01156-16] [PMID: 27572398]

[58]   Shannon A, Selisko B, Le N, *et al.* Favipiravir strikes the SARS-CoV-2 at its Achilles heel, the RNA polymerase. 2020.bioRxiv [PREPRINT]
[http://dx.doi.org/10.1101/2020.05.15.098731]

[59]   Furuta Y, Gowen BB, Takahashi K, Shiraki K, Smee DF, Barnard DL. Favipiravir (T-705), a novel viral RNA polymerase inhibitor. Antiviral Res 2013; 100(2): 446-54.

[http://dx.doi.org/10.1016/j.antiviral.2013.09.015] [PMID: 24084488]

[60]   Furuta Y, Takahashi K, Fukuda Y, *et al. In vitro* and *in vivo* activities of anti-influenza virus compound T-705. Antimicrob Agents Chemother 2002; 46(4): 977-81.
[http://dx.doi.org/10.1128/AAC.46.4.977-981.2002] [PMID: 11897578]

[61]   Jochmans D, van Nieuwkoop S, Smits SL, Neyts J, Fouchier RAM, van den Hoogen BG. Anti-viral activity of favipiravir (T-705) against a broad range of paramyxoviruses *in vitro* and against human metapneumovirus in hamsters. Antimicrob Agents Chemother 2016; 60(8): 4620-9.
[http://dx.doi.org/10.1128/AAC.00709-16] [PMID: 27185803]

[62]   Wang M, Cao R, Zhang L, *et al.* Remdesivir and chloroquine effectively inhibit the recently emerged novel coronavirus (2019-nCoV) *in vitro.* Cell Res 2020; 30(3): 269-71. a
[http://dx.doi.org/10.1038/s41422-020-0282-0] [PMID: 32020029]

[63]   Choy KT, Wong AYL, Kaewpreedee P, *et al.* Remdesivir, lopinavir, emetine, and homoharringtonine inhibit SARS-CoV-2 replication *in vitro.* Antiviral Res 2020; 178: 104786.
[http://dx.doi.org/10.1016/j.antiviral.2020.104786] [PMID: 32251767]

[64]   Pizzorno A, Padey B, Dubois J, *et al. In vitro* evaluation of antiviral activity of single and combined repurposable drugs against SARS-CoV-2. Antiviral Res 2020; 181: 104878.
[http://dx.doi.org/10.1016/j.antiviral.2020.104878] [PMID: 32679055]

[65]   Streeter DG, Witkowski JT, Khare GP, *et al.* Mechanism of action of 1- -D-ribofuranosyl-1,- ,4-triazole-3-carboxamide (Virazole), a new broad-spectrum antiviral agent. Proc Natl Acad Sci USA 1973; 70(4): 1174-8.
[http://dx.doi.org/10.1073/pnas.70.4.1174] [PMID: 4197928]

[66]   Wray SK, Gilbert BE, Noall MW, Knight V. Mode of action of ribavirin: Effect of nucleotide pool alterations on influenza virus ribonucleoprotein synthesis. Antiviral Res 1985; 5(1): 29-37.
[http://dx.doi.org/10.1016/0166-3542(85)90012-9] [PMID: 3985606]

[67]   Crance JM, Scaramozzino N, Jouan A, Garin D. Interferon, ribavirin, 6-azauridine and glycyrrhizin: antiviral compounds active against pathogenic flaviviruses. Antiviral Res 2003; 58(1): 73-9.
[http://dx.doi.org/10.1016/S0166-3542(02)00185-7] [PMID: 12719009]

[68]   Cinatl J, Morgenstern B, Bauer G, Chandra P, Rabenau H, Doerr HW. Glycyrrhizin, an active component of liquorice roots, and replication of SARS-associated coronavirus. Lancet 2003; 361(9374): 2045-6.
[http://dx.doi.org/10.1016/S0140-6736(03)13615-X] [PMID: 12814717]

[69]   Dey SK, Saini M, Dhembla C, *et al.* Suramin, Penciclovir and Anidulafungin bind nsp12, which governs the RNA-dependent-RNA polymerase activity of SARS-CoV-2, with higher interaction energy than Remdesivir, indicating potential in the treatment of Covid-19 infection. 2020.OSF Preprints [PREPRINT]
[http://dx.doi.org/10.31219/osf.io/urxwh]

[70]   Kumar S, Zhi K, Mukherji A, Gerth K. Repurposing anti-viral protease inhibitors using extracellular vesicles for potential therapy of COVID-19. Viruses 2020; 12(5): 486.
[http://dx.doi.org/10.3390/v12050486] [PMID: 32357553]

[71]   Lee C. Griffithsin, a highly potent broad-spectrum anti-viral lectin from red algae: from discovery to clinical application. Mar Drugs 2019; 17(10): 567.
[http://dx.doi.org/10.3390/md17100567] [PMID: 31590428]

[72]   Lin MH, Moses DC, Hsieh CH, *et al.* Disulfiram can inhibit MERS and SARS coronavirus papain-like proteases *via* different modes. Antiviral Res 2018; 150: 155-63.
[http://dx.doi.org/10.1016/j.antiviral.2017.12.015] [PMID: 29289665]

[73]   Xu Z, Peng C, Shi Y, *et al.* Nelfinavir was predicted to be a potential inhibitor of 2019; BioRxiv 2020.01.27.921627.

[74]   Chen H, Zhang Z, Wang L, *et al.* First clinical study using HCV protease inhibitor danoprevir to treat

naive and experienced COVID-19patients. MedRxiv 2020; 2020.03.22.20034041.

[75]   Westover JB, Mathis A, Taylor R, *et al.* Galidesivir limits Rift Valley fever virus infection and disease in Syrian golden hamsters. Antiviral Res 2018; 156: 38-45.
       [http://dx.doi.org/10.1016/j.antiviral.2018.05.013] [PMID: 29864447]

[76]   Liu J, Cao R, Xu M, *et al.* Hydroxychloroquine, a less toxic derivative of chloroquine, is effective in inhibiting SARS-CoV-2 infection *in vitro.* Cell Discov 2020; 6(1): 16.
       [http://dx.doi.org/10.1038/s41421-020-0156-0] [PMID: 32194981]

[77]   Ghanbari R, Teimoori A, Sadeghi A, *et al.* Existing antiviral options against SARS-CoV-2 replication in COVID-19 patients. Future Microbiol 2020; 15(18): 1747-58.
       [http://dx.doi.org/10.2217/fmb-2020-0120] [PMID: 33404263]

CHAPTER 4

Targeting the Viral Entry Pathways through Repurposed Drugs in Sars-Cov-2 Infection

Manisha Mulchandani[1], Amit Kumar Palai[1], Anjali Bhosale[1], Farhan Mazahir[1] and Awesh K. Yadav[1,*]

[1] *Department of Pharmaceutics, National Institute of Pharmaceutical Education and Research (NIPER) Raebareli, Lucknow, Uttar Pradesh, India*

Abstract: SARS-CoV-2 belongs to the family coronviradae and the disease caused by this virus is known as COVID-19. Viral entry into the cell is favored by spike glycoprotein, which interacts with Angiotensin-converting-enzyme-2 (ACE-2). Moreover, proteins such as Transmembrane Protease Serine-2 (TMPRSS-2), are responsible for viral fusion with cellular epithelium. Traditional drug discovery methods and their development process are time-consuming as well as expensive. Thus, there is a need for a method that can overcome such drawbacks. Drug repurposing is an approach in which we can use an existing drug that is already being used for another disease. The repurposing of drugs is also known as repositioning. It is the process that identifies new therapeutic use for existing or available drugs. Hydroxychloroquine inhibits ACE-2 glycosylation virus entry to the host body; arbidol prevents fusion of viral lipid shell with cell membrane hence restricting contact and penetration of virus. Drug repurposing could be a successful strategy for the treatment of sporadic, neglected diseases, difficult-to-treat diseases, and the current pandemic situation, *i.e.*, COVID-19. However, there is no denying the fact that there are several limitations to this approach.

keywords: Animal model, Antiviral, Computational approach, COVID-19, Drug repurposing, Experimental approach, Phytochemicals, SARS-CoV-2 Spike Protein, Viral inhibition.

INTRODUCTION

COVID-19 is caused by the infection of SARS-CoV-2 (severe acute respiratory syndrome coronavirus 2). This virus belongs to the Nidovirales order family coronviradae and has two subfamilies, Coronavirinae and Torovirinae. As the name suggests, it affects the respiratory system mainly. This virus spread like a

---

* **Corresponding Author Awesh K Yadav:** Department of Pharmaceutics, National Institute of Pharmaceutical Education and Research, (NIPER) Raebareli, A Transit Campus at Bijnor-Sisendi Road, Near CRPF Base Camp, Sarojini Nagar, Lucknow, Uttar Pradesh-226002, India; Tel: +918989154900;
E-mail: awesh.yadav@niperraebareli.edu.in

Tabish Qidwai (Ed.)

fire in the jungle worldwide and became a pandemic leading to multiple infections and several deaths occur due to this virus. The general symptoms of people infected with SARS-CoV-2 are cough, chest discomfort, dyspnea (Which occurs in the majority of people), and symptoms that are related to gastrointestinal discomforts like vomiting and diarrhea (Which occur rarely). The immune system also gets affected; there will be a decrease in the lymphocyte count. It affects the major vital organs of the body lungs, heart, and kidneys. It is found that people infected with SARS-CoV-2 showed glassy opacity in the lungs. In clinical chemistry, it is found that there is an increase in the alanine transaminase, lactate dehydrogenase, and D- dimer count [1, 2].

Viral entry is by various proteins and enzymes (Figs. **1** and **2**). The envelope-embedded surface-located spike (S) glycoprotein is responsible for coronavirus entrance. Most of the time, host proteases will cleave this S protein into the S1 and S2 subunits, which are important for receptor identification and membrane fusion. S1 is further separated into two parts: an N-terminal domain (NTD) and a C-terminal domain (CTD), both of which serve as receptor-binding entrance points. SARS-CoV and MERS-CoV, for example, use the S1 CTD to detect receptors (also called receptor binding domain). The spike protein of SARS-CoV-2 interacts with the Angiotensin-converting-enzyme-2 (ACE-2) receptor of the host cell (S). ACE-2 is an enzyme that breaks down the bigger protein angiotensinogen to produce tiny proteins that control cell activity. Angiotensin II (ANG II) can cause inflammation and the death of cells in the alveoli, which are important for delivering oxygen to the body; ACE-2 counteracts these negative effects of ANG II. The SARS-CoV-2 virus attaches to ACE-2 stops it from regulating ANG II signaling. As a result, the activity of ACE-2 is blocked, erasing the gaps in ANG II signaling and allowing more ANG II to reach injured tissues. In covid19 patients, this reduced breaking is expected to harm the lungs and heart. Another enzyme such as Transmembrane Prot Transmembrane Protease Serine-2 (TMPRSS-2) is encoded by the TMPRSS-2 gene in humans. TMPRSS-2 is a cell surface protein produced largely by endothelial cells in the respiratory and gastrointestinal systems. It functions as a serine protease, cleaving peptide bonds in proteins with serine as the nucleophilic amino acid at the active site. SARS-CoV-2 and other coronaviruses require TMPRSS-2 to enter the body. By binding to ACE-2, TMPRSS-2 activates the spike protein domain (a glycoprotein present on coronaviruses), causing the virus to fuse to the respiratory epithelia on the cell surface in case of non-endocytic entry. Cathepsin L is a cysteine protease that shows its best activity in a slightly acidic medium. Without cleavage of spike protein by this protease, the virus can not enter the cell; this process occurs when the virus follows endocytic entry. In addition, refer to Table **1** for brief information regarding the various variants of SARS-CoV-2.

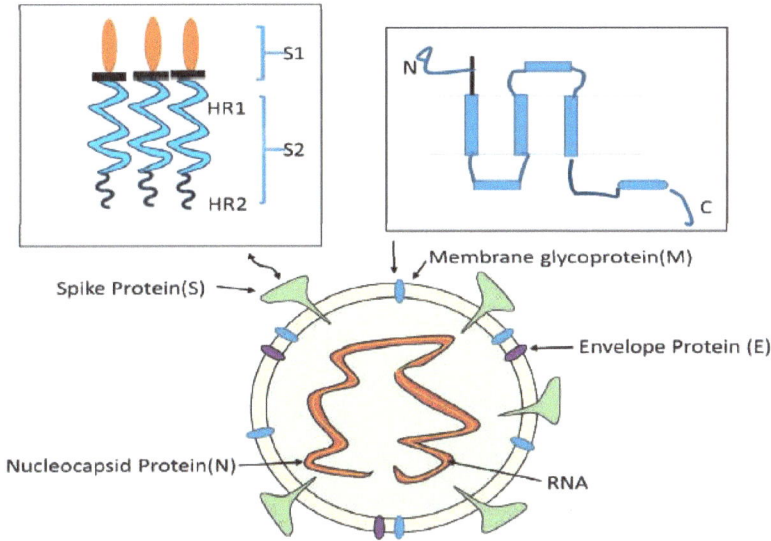

Fig. (1). Illustration of SARS-CoV-2 biological structure. S proteins of the coronavirus from their crown-like appearance. S proteins are cleaved by furin or related enzyme into S1 and S2 subunits in the Golgi complex region. The M-protein is composed of three parts, a short N-terminal domain (situated outside the particle), three transmembrane domains, and a carboxy domain (situated inside the particle).

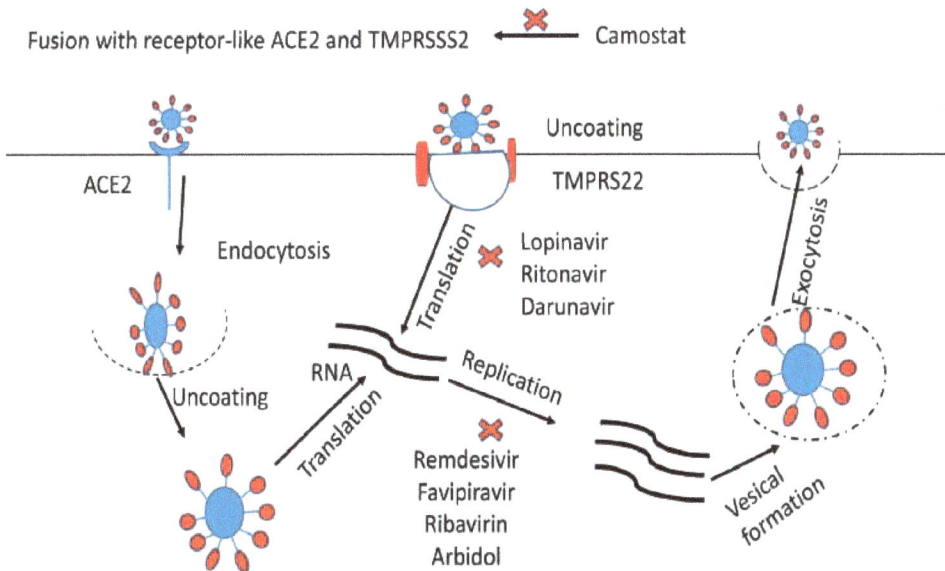

Fig. (2). Illustration of the mechanism of virus uptake inhibition by various repurposed drugs.

Table 1. List of various variants of SARS-CoV-2 identified during the COVID-19 pandemic.

Variant Name	First Identified	Country in which the First Case Detected	References
Alpha	September 2020	United Kingdom	[3]
Beta	May 2020	South Africa	
Gamma	November 2020	South America	
Delta	October 2020	Asia (Counties like India, Bangladesh, Malaysia, and Myanmar)	
Eta	December 2020	Nigeria and United Kingdom	
Lotta	November 2020	New York (USA)	
Kappa	October 2020	India	
Lambda	December 2020	Peru	

Keeping in mind the current situation, it is obvious that the existing drug can be of great help. As their safety profile is previously defined, it can be used rapidly for treatment. Drug repurposing utilizes various approaches for selecting the best candidate, which include computational and experimental approaches. The computational approach includes machine learning which combines molecular docking studies, metabolic data, and its resemblance to SARS-CoV-2; GWAS (Genome-Wide Association Studies) can also help study drug resemblance with disease conditions. Other studies like AI (Artificial Intelligence) based learning, signature-based studies, *etc.*, which are tough at the initial stage, have a lot of potential in finding the better candidate for drug repurposing. An experimental approach includes target-based, binding-based, drug-centric, and phenotype-based techniques for drug repurposing. Mostly these approaches focus on the effect of the drug candidate on the diseases. Drugs such as arbidol prevent the fusion of viral lipid shell with the cell membrane, and hydroxychloroquine inhibits ACE-2 glycosylation virus entry to the cell body; camostat mesylate, a protease inhibitor inhibits TMPRSS-2 protein, thus restricting the spike protein activation and preventing fusion of the virus to the cellular epithelium, remdesivir interferes exoribonuclease leading to disruption of RNA. Many other drugs have been used in SARS-CoV-2 as repurposed candidates, such as favipiravir, lopinavir, darunavir, tocilizumab, ritonavir, ribavirin, and interferons.

DRUG REPURPOSING

It is an approach in which we can use an existing drug already in use for another disease, like hydroxychloroquine used, for the treatment of malaria, but it has also been used at the time of the COVID-19 Pandemic. We can use that same drug for our purpose or any other disease; this concept is termed the repurposing of drugs. This approach is economical and efficient, and the results of the study can be approved in minimum time and are highly cost-effective, compared with the cost to develop a new drug. The motive of drug repurposing is to identify a new clinical use for the drugs which are proven to be safe as well as effective in clinical trials, and these can be approved for treatment for other diseases also reduced for the manufacturing of new drugs, with significant time saving and to speed up the traditional process of drug discovery. From this strategy, the cost is preclinical as well as clinical trials. The repurposed drugs come into four categories (i) therapeutic assets with residual patent life but then are not permitted for human use, (ii) therapeutics which are having residual patent life that is recently being used for more than one indication but can also be used for the treatment of other diseases, (iii) therapeutic which are having no patent life that is not recently being sold because they were either not permitted or were withdrawn, (iv) those therapeutics which are having no patent life recently developed by generic companies and permitted for certain indications as well as available by prescription from healthcare suppliers; based on the discovery of new therapeutic uses for existing drugs. If the repurposing drugs are to be distributed to the public, they must meet all the normal benefit-risk assessment requirements. They must be safe, effective, and qualitative. All drug regulatory agencies are teamed up through the international council of medicines regulatory authorities (ICMRA), and these are committed to fast-moving regulations. All major agencies like the United Kingdom, the United States, Japan, and Europe already have robust procedures in place for accelerated approvals because they require minimal evidence. For example, remdesivir is a repurposed drug initially being used for Ebola. In the Japanese authorization, remdesivir is under the exceptional approval pathway; in the USA, emergency use approval and the United Kingdom access were granted within a short period to medicine [4 - 6]. Refer to Table **2**.

Drug Repurposed for COVID-19 – Drugs such as favipiravir, remdesivir, hydroxychloroquine, lopinavir, darunavir, tocilizumab, ritonavir, atazanavir, ribavirin arbidol these drugs are found to have inhibitory effects on the viral structure [7]. Refer to Figs. (**2** and **3**).

Remdesivir

It is a prodrug that gets converted intracellularly in its adenosine triphosphate form. Remdesevir has a broad-spectrum antiviral activity that is effective in various viral diseases like Ebola and can inhibit RNA-dependent RNA polymerase. Coronavirus has proofreading capacity. This drug can interfere with the proofreading enzyme, which is exoribonuclease which corrects any error present in the RNA, ultimately leading to RNA disruption. This drug is a nucleoside analog, having great antiviral action. The *in-vivo* study suggested that the drug is used to lower the chances of lung infection. Up to 200 mg dose can be administered intravenously. General adverse effects like nausea, respiratory failure, and GIT problems (*i.e.*, constipation) have been reported [8].

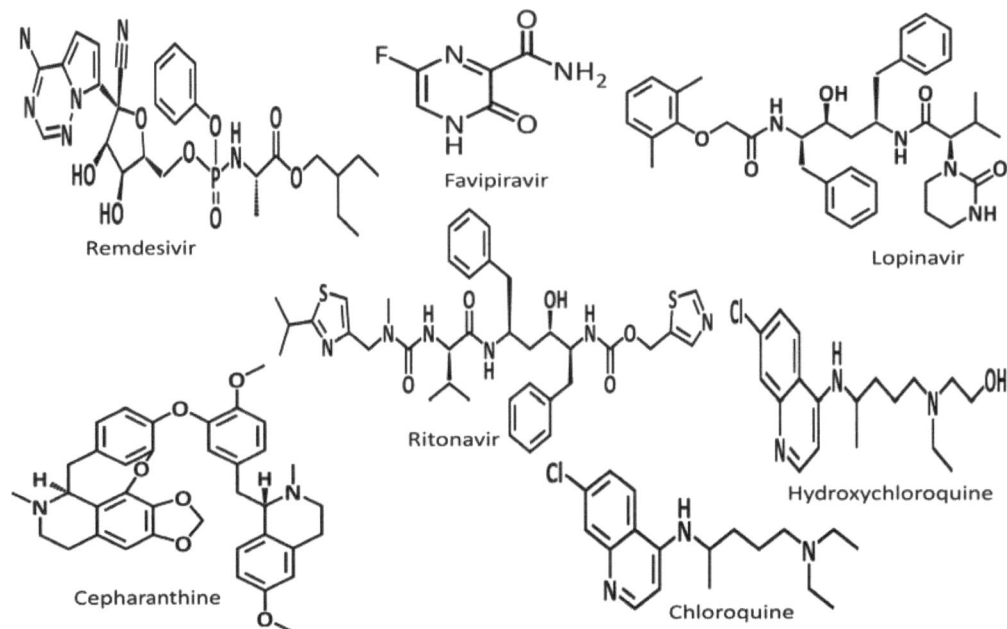

Fig. (3). Representation of the chemical structure of different repurposed drug candidates.

Favipiravir

This drug is being used for the treatment of influenza in many countries. Like remdesvir is also an RNA-dependent RNA polymerase inhibitor and can be administered to the patient by oral route. Favipiravir is an example of a prodrug, and a purine analog gets converted into its active phosphorylated form, producing its therapeutic effects. The phosphorylated form directly inhibits the influenza virus's RNA-dependent RNA polymerase. This drug has broad-spectrum antiviral activity. Results obtained after *in-vivo* studies in Guinea pigs suggested no evidence of potential toxicity after receiving a 500mg dose of the Favipiravir [9].

Lopinavir and Ritonavir

These drugs are protease inhibitors administered in combination to increase the half-life of lopinavir. These drugs are already used in the treatment of HIV-1. *In vitro* studies have shown that the drugs are effective in SARS-CoV-2. Lopinavir and Ritonavir can also use along with the interferons and have shown great efficacy in the treatment of MERS. The common adverse effects of using these drugs are nausea and diarrhea. They can use with other relevant therapies [10].

Hydroxychloroquine and Chloroquine

These drugs are already in use for the treatment of malaria, and rheumatoid arthritis, and can act as an anti-inflammatory agents. It works by raising the pH of the endosome, changing the pH outside of the optimum range, thereby indirectly inhibiting cathepsin protease activity. These drugs have an affinity to sialic acid receptors and inhibit the ACE2 glycosylation virus entry to the host body. Chloroquine shows more toxicity than hydroxychloroquine, whereas hydroxychloroquine should be administered to the patient with liver and kidney dysfunctions *via* the precautions route [11, 12].

Tocilizumab

It is a monoclonal antibody as it has been found that there is a cytokinin storm in the COVID-19 infection which will cause an increase in the level of IL-6 (interleukin-6). The levels of interleukin-6 are generally higher in severely ill patients. Hence, tocilizumab is used to control the IL-6 levels. This drug is already used in the treatment of rheumatoid arthritis for the long term with some limited side effects. It shows few adverse effects, *i.e.*, liver toxicity, steatosis, headache, and nausea [13].

Darunavir

This drug is being prescribed for the treatment of HIV, and it's a protease inhibitor. This drug has better effects with fewer numbers of side effects. The drug can make an enzyme-inhibitor complex. Its structure helps in the binding, making it more effective than other drugs of the protease inhibitor category. This drug should be used with precautions in patients suffering from cardiac problems [14].

Ribavirin

This is a guanosine analog and can inhibit the replication of both DNA as well as RNA. This drug inhibits the RNA polymerase and alters the capping, leading to RNA damage. It also inhibits the mechanism responsible for the generation of guanosine in the body. This drug is already used in the treatment of hepatitis. A dose of 500 mg, 2-3 times a day, along with lopinavir and ritonavir, can be recommended. Hemolytic anemia has been reported as the most common adverse effect after the administration of Ribavirin [15].

Arbidol

This drug is derived from indole and can be used against enveloped as well as non-enveloped viruses. This drug is currently being used to treat influenza A & B, and hepatitis C viruses. can also be an effective option for treatment for SARS-CoV-2. The administration of arbidol, along with lopinavir and ritonavir, was found to inhibit the development of pulmonary lesions [16].

Camostat Mesylate

S1/S2' and S2' are cleavage sites on the Te SARS-CoV-2 Spike protein. The furin proprotein convertase is principally responsible for cleaving the S1/S2' site for non-endocytic entry. This cleavage might then aid in revealing the S2' site to surface trypsin-like serine proteases like TMPRSS2. The S2' site is just upstream of the fusion peptide (FP), and TMPRSS2 cleaves it, exposing the hydrophobic peptide (FP) for membrane insertion. TMPRSS2 protein inhibitor helps in the priming of the spike protein of SARS-CoV-2, and this drug can block the TMPRSS2 protein. One of the first small chemical inhibitors to be proven to have significant effectiveness in preventing SARS-CoV-2 entrance into cells was camostat. This drug comes under the category of protease inhibitor. The *in-vivo* studies indicated that the drug is effective in decreasing mortality. It is also found that 600mg twice a day is effective against the treatment of COVID-19 [17].

Nafamostat

It is an anticoagulant as well as a serine protease inhibitor and is used to inhibit the entry of viruses inside the epithelial cells by preventing the fusion of membranes and decreasing the release of cathepsin B. The more powerful counterpart, nafamostat, has been proven to stop SARS-CoV-2 multiplication in Calu-3 cells. This drug has been found effective for the treatment of acute pancreatitis and is used in MERS (Middle East Respiratory Syndrome). *In-vitro* studies are done in E6 cells and found that this drug is effective against SARS-CoV-2 [18].

Sofosbuvir

This prodrug converts into its phosphorylated form to inhibit RNA-dependent RNA polymerase. Generally, it is used in the treatment of Hepatitis C. It is also being used along with ledipasvir to treat viral hepatitis. Also, docking studies were carried out to evaluate the effectiveness of the sofosbuvir against COVID-19. Sofosbuvir can be tolerated up to 400mg/daily [19, 20].

Cepharanthine

This drug is of natural origin and obtained from *Stephania cepharantha*. It is an alkaloid and possesses several properties like anti-inflammatory and anti-viral activities. It can inhibit the entry of the virus at low doses. This drug is also recommended for the treatment of Alopecia as well as leukopenia and can decrease the viral RNA load [21].

Nelfinavir

This drug is used as an HIV-Protease inhibitor and inhibits the replication of SARS-CoV-2. This drug, along with other antiretroviral drugs, is suggested to treat HIV infection. This drug can be the more superior to other protease inhibitors due to its inability to prevent replication. Molecular docking-based analysis has shown that this drug is effective against SARS-CoV-2 [22].

Fluoxetine

Fluoxetine is a selective serotonin reuptake inhibitor used as an anti-depressant, for premenstrual dysphoric disorder and pain disorders. It is believed that SARS-CoV-2 activates the ceramide system. As SARS-CoV-2 cleaves the sphingomyelin and converts it into a highly lipophilic substance ceramide which serves as a platform to enter the cell. and this system is altered by fluoxetine. This helps in the prevention of SARS-CoV-2 replication [23].

Enfuvirtide

Enfuvirtide is a fusion inhibitor that has been authorised to treat HIV infection. However, viral fusion with the cellular membrane might be a therapeutic target. As both HR1 and HR2 are required to generate the 6HB and subsequently fuse, developing a peptide that mimics one area will compete with the development of the fusion core. Other viruses having heptad regions, such as HIV, have been prevented from entering using this method. Hence, it can be used in the case of SARS-Cov-2 [24].

Table 2. Repurposed along with their mechanism of action.

Drug	Mechanism	Uses	References
Remdesivir	RNA dependent RNA polymerase inhibitor	Antiviral Drug	[25]
Favipiravir	RNA dependent RNA polymerase inhibitor	Antiviral Drug	[26]
Lopinavir and Ritonavir	Protease Inhibitor	HIV-1 virus	[10]
Hydroxychloroquine and Chloroquine	Inhibit ACE2 Glycosylation	Malaria and Rheumatoid Arthritis	[27]
Tocilizumab	Interaleukin-6 inhibitor	Rheumatoid Arthritis	[28]
Darunavir	Protease Inhibitor	HIV	[29]

(Table 2) cont.....

Drug	Mechanism	Uses	References
Ribavirin	RNA polymerase inhibitor	Hepatitis	[30]
Arbidol	Inhibits cellular entry	Influenza A and B	[31]
Camostat Mesylate	TMPRSS2 protein inhibitor	Chronic Pancreatitis	[32]
Nafamostat	Inhibit cellular entry	Acute Pancreatitis.	[33]
Sofosbuvir	RNA-dependent RNA polymerase inhibitor	Hepatitis C	[34]
Cepharanthine	Inhibits cellular entry	Alopecia	[35]
Nelfinavir	Protease Inhibitor	HIV	[36]

Role of Phytochemicals

SARS, MERS, influenza, and dengue virus symptoms have all been treated with antiviral herbal medications in the past. Secondary plant metabolites may affect viral replication at one or more stages. Anxiety and other upper respiratory symptoms linked with COVID-19 may be alleviated by herbal medicines with significant antioxidant and antiviral action. To combat the SARS-CoV-2 pandemic, researchers used computational, *in-vitro*, and *in-vivo* investigations to look into the potential of therapeutic plants and natural products. In January 2020, Wang *et al.* Conducted retrospective research at Shanghai Public Health Clinical Center, China, on four confirmed COVID-19 patients to assess the effect of a combination of Shufeng Jiedu Capsule (SFJDC), traditional Chinese medicine, arbidol, and lopinavir/ritonavir. In the most recent edition of Diagnosis and Treatment of Pneumonia Caused by 2019-nCoV, SFJDC is also indicated for treating COVID-19 infection. The findings were promising and warranted more investigation. Zhang and colleagues conducted a logical *in silico* screening of certain prospective of Chinese herbal medicines to find medicinal plants and phytochemicals that might directly suppress the growth of cancer cells. These include quercetin, kaempferol, betulinic acid, coumaryltyramine, crytptotanshinone, sugiol, and other compounds. Forsythiae fructus, Mori cortex, Liquorice, Ardisia japonicae herba, Eriobotryae folium, and other Chinese herbal plants that may contain these ingredients can be used to treat respiratory disorders. Qamar *et al.* searched a medicinal plant database with 32,297 putative anti-viral phytochemicals/traditional Chinese medicinal compounds and chose the best hits that might reduce SARS-CoV-2 3CLpro activity and thereby virus multiplication. Phytochemicals such as 5,7,3',4'-Tetrahydroxy2'-(3,3dimethylallyl)isoflavone from Psorothamnus sarborescens, Myricitrin from Myrica cerifera, Methyl rosmarinate from Hyptisa trorubens Poit, Calceolarioside B from Fraxinus sieboldiana, and Licoleafol from Glycyrrhiza uralensis were included and concluded that these phytochemicals might be used as anti-COVID-19 lead compounds in the creation of new drugs to treat COVID-19.Scutellaria baicalensis (Family: Lamiaceae) is a Chinese medicinal plant whose roots have been shown to have significant antiviral action against the coronavirus family. Both Baicalein and baicalin are responsible for the antiviral action of the plant. These two natural compounds have antiviral properties, blocking dengue virus entrance into the host and limiting virus multiplication [22]. Baicalin, according to Zhang and Liu, might be employed as a therapeutic option to boost immunity. Quercetin is a flavonoid that has five hydroxyl groups present in Allium cepa, Ginkgo biloba, Sambucus canadensis, and Hypericum perforatum has been shown to prevent the H5N1 virus from entering the body in its early stages. It has a stronger inhibitory effect on Angiotensin-Converting Enzyme than rutin, kaempferol, rhoifolin, and apigenin K flavonoids, as seen by their IC50 values. Nigella sativa may have the necessary potency to be utilized as a COVID-19 complementary and alternative medicine. Its bioactive components, particularly thymoquinone, have been shown to have antiviral properties. They went on to say that as thymoquinone is a smaller hydrophobic molecule that it can attach itself to the lipophilic part of the virus and oxidize it, Thus having a lethal effect on the virus. In contrast, Rahman theorized that thymoquinone and nigellimine may prevent SARS-CoV-2 from infecting pneumocytes *via* the Angiotensin-converting enzyme 2 (ACE2) pathway. The researcher also suggested that zinc supplementation might boost black seed's antiviral activity against COVID-19. In the presence of thymoquinone and other bioactive chemicals that serve as ionophores, Zinc absorption into pneumocytes would be improved, which will not only hinder the reproduction of new viral entities by inhibiting RdRp but also encourage host immunity. Al-Noaemi also advised co-administering Nigella sativa with hydroxychloroquine (HCQ) as an adjuvant treatment to minimize toxicity and enhance HCQ's antiviral effects against COVID-19. Mpiana and colleagues believe that Aloe vera extract has abundant zinc in it, as well as its secondary bioactive metabolites, which could be used to treat COVID-19 because of its ability to decrease the development of proinflammatory action. In the Democratic Republic of the Congo, the Aloe vera plant is identified as a promising nominee for SARS-CoV-2 treatment. Its extract, as well as its bioactive components, anthraquinones, have been proven in several investigations to exhibit good broad-spectrum virucidal activity. Zinc, which is found in aloe vera, has been shown to prevent the reproduction of retroviruses such as SARS-CoV-2. Using an artificial method, Gyebi and colleagues evaluated 62 alkaloids and 100 terpenoid bioactive natural compounds obtained from native African herbs as possible inhibitors of coronavirus 3-chymotrypsin-like protease (3CLpro). They suggested that *in-vivo* studies be conducted to assess the therapeutic effectiveness of 10-Hydroxyusambarensine, Cryptoquindoline, 6-Oxoisoiguesterin, and 22-Hydroxyhopan-3-one against SARS-CoV-2 3CLpro. In a computer simulation, isothymol, a prominent ingredient that contributes to around 51% of Ammoides verticillata plants was discovered to decrease the angiotensin-converting enzyme 2 (ACE2) receptor. It forms a stable contact with the ACE-2 receptor, according to a molecular docking study. Glycyrrhetinic acid, Glycyrrhizin, and bioactive ingredients of liquorice can increase nitrous oxide synthase, preventing viral multiplication, according to the study's findings. Because of its expectorant and antitussive properties, liquorice root may give symptomatic relief to COVID-19 patients who are suffering from dyspnea. The anti-reverse transcriptase activity of Vitex negundo (Chinese chaste tree) and Solanum nigrum (Black nightshade) might be exploited for COVID-19 drug screening and development. In Chinese traditional medicine, elderberry, self-healing, and peacock flowers are used to treat cold, cough, and flu symptoms. These herbs should be investigated further, as some of them may have the potential to be a remedy against COVID-19 due to their ability to boost immunity, and antioxidants and decrease inflammatory responses [37].

DRUGS REPURPOSING APPROACHES

There are 3 steps to be followed for drug repurposing, including identifying perfect candidates for drug repurposing, evaluating and studying the biological, chemical, and behavioral responses for the drug in the model, and other studies defining the preclinical studies. Then the evaluation of efficacy studies of candidate drugs should be directed to phase-II of the clinical trials. The systematic approach for determining the repurposing of the drug can be divided into 2 groups (1) Computational Approach (2) Experimental Approach. Refer to Figs. (4-6).

Computational Approach: following are the types of computational approaches:

Machine Learning-Based

It includes a detailed study of various genomics, proteomics transcriptomes, molecular docking studies, metabolomics data, chemical structure, and past clinical data regarding SARS-CoV-2 and MERS-CoV; these can help us to figure out the best candidate for repurposing of the drug against SARS-CoV-2. Various Machine Learning (MLs) techniques and methods, such as deep learning and neural network, were applied to sorting out the drug candidate for repurposing. Deep learning algorithms are used to determine the interaction between drugs and proteins and the binding affinity between them. For example, Beck and colleagues utilized MT-DTI (Molecule Transformer-Drug Target Interaction) model on atazanavir to determine its inhabitation activity against SARS-CoV-2-like proteinase (Diss.constant-94) [38]. Numerous ML methods collectively have helped in sorting out around 41 drugs as repurposable candidates, and some of the drugs can back up by the existing clinical data related to proteomics and transcriptomics [39]. Though approved drugs exist, various ML methods are

virtual screening helped in identifying novel compounds such as anti HCV drug IDX-IS4 can be proven to be effective against SARS-CoV-2 [40]. Other methods include generating a neural network, which could help in easing out the methods for drug repurposing against COVID-19 treatment where the nodes represent various biomedical entities, including drugs, protein, and disease in which the edges of it signify the disease's protein interaction. By this method, Hsieh and Coworkers found around 22 drugs and various drug combinations regarding COVID-19 treatment [41]. ML methods are heavily based on the multiple sources of data included as these methods, in general, are quite sensitive depending on the type and quality, and quantity of data set. Moreover, COVID-19 emerged in late 19, so there is no availability of extensive studies regarding the data to be included, the behavior, and the types of data to be included during the studies. This results in different inferences drawn depending on the data included, which may affect the methods of choosing a perfect drug repurposing candidate. Hence, there is a lack of reliable predictions, which is a drawback of the MLS methods. To avoid this, researchers must focus on determining a better algorithm that can keep up with the current situation and should have a better scope of evolving with time.

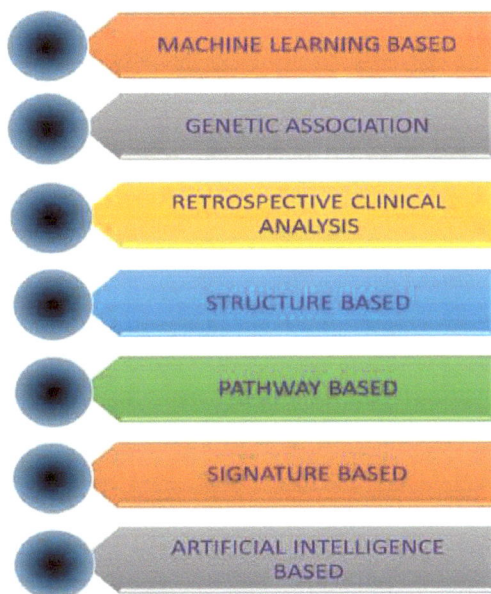

Fig. (4). Types of the computational approach.

Genetic Association

Genome-wide association studies (GWAS) would help determine the genetic variant of various infectious diseases. Its increased hold on the biological data would help in perfectly determining novel targets for drug repurposing. The data obtained from the GWAS study on 1980 ill COVID-19 patients suggested that the 3P21.31 gene cluster is the genetic susceptibility loss in most patients with COVID-19, *i.e.*, in case of repurposing failure [42]. This gene cluster of 3P21.31 consists of SLC6A20, LZTFLI, CCR9, FYCOL, CSCRS, and XCR-1; these genes can serve as target genes for the treatment of COVID-19. Though the GWAS study bestowed us various repurposing opportunities, its association with huge data makes maintenance and proper analysis tedious. For this reason, they are to be investigated by orthogonal methods. Secondly, multiple testing problem is associated with GWAS due to insufficiency of genome present, which can be well encountered by the collaboration of clinicians and researchers. Cryptic population stratification poses another problem in GWAS. Family-based GWAS or population substructure correction approaches should be undertaken by the researchers [43].

Retrospecting Clinical Analysis

The enormous success stories of retrospective clinical analysis are equally encouraging, for example famous "Blue pill" sildenafil. Sildenafil is a PDE-5 inhibitor whose main purpose of development is to treat angina pectoris. The phase-I clinical trial has shown dilation of blood vessels in the penis [44]. So though it was not able to treat angina successfully later, it was rescued and repurposed for treatment of erectile dysfunctions. Drugs such as propranolol used in osteoporosis and melanoma treatment of breast cancer using raloxifene and metformin are all among various success stories of drug repurposing using retrospective clinical analysis. Hence, it was wise to apply this boon during the pandemic against COVID-19, and it has proved to be fruitful. Using this method, various candidates such as melatonin carvedilol [45] and Umifenavir [46], hydroxyl chloroquine, and drug combination such as Oseltamavir in combination with hydroxyl chloroquine has shown the potential for treating diseases which are confirmed by retrospective comparison. This method is not only used for drug repurposing but also provides a new threshold for the failed drugs to be rescued and reused in the different therapeutic applications, and can serve as the better standard for competition in the market, through ample data sources such as Vigibase (WHO base for ADR), and FAERS (FDA adverse event reporting system). Both the data, including data from clinical trials and post-marketing surveillance data, are available, but the major problem is posed by patient confidentiality, legal difficulties, and limited research capability.

Structure-Based

For COVID-19, a mainly target-centric approach is preferred due to the rich sources of data obtained from the studies conducted on SARS-CoV-2 and MERS-CoV and cellular targets. These studies have helped us in identifying a particular target area, and focusing our attention on implicating various drugs towards the target is the prime approach example, ACE2; Elfiky used target based centric approach against the virus by usual molecular docking method on SARS-CoV-2 RNA depending on RNA polymerase (RdRp), and found that various antiviral drugs like ribavirin, remdesivir, sofosbuvir, galdesivir and tenofovir serve as inhibitors of RdRP, with -7.0 to -7.8Kcal/mol (binding energy) [47]. Another way includes an antiviral target-based drug-centric approach, which is used for determining potential targets for COVID-19 through molecular docking. For example, Martin and Cheng found toremifene as a good candidate for Covid treatment, and the molecular target of it was found to be spike glycoprotein and NSP14 [48]. In the host target based target centric approach, Khelfaoui *et al.* utilized the finding that ACE2 along with spike glycoprotein of SARS-CoV-2 helped the entry of virus and used a drug bank database to find out which drug has a high affinity for binding to ACE2 and SARS–COV-2 spike glycoprotein/ ACE-2 complex by molecular docking method [49]. From the studies, it was concluded that delapril, ramipril and lisinopril show better affinity to ACE-2 and spike ACE-2 complex. Various online databases like GHDDI, COVID-19 information-sharing portal, and Covid scholar are available. There are various disadvantages associated with the structure-based approach. First of all, it aims at a single protein or gene, which is a simplistic approach to disease progression. In a disease progression, various factors are responsible, and treating a single target can't be of much help. Moreover, most of the screening done in this method is in a cell-free system, so chances are there that the hit selected can pose various threats like cytotoxicity, decreased bioavailability, shelf life, *etc.* So a better *in-vitro* approach is needed.

Pathway Based

The mechanism of this method is quite self-explanatory. In this method, the metabolic pathways, the interaction between the proteins, and data obtained from different gene expression studies are taken into consideration to determine the target for drug repurposing. The main drawback of pathway mapping is that it is not an independent process; it largely depends upon gene annotation. The problem with gene annotation is that it is not complete and would not be available for the next few years and the existing genes require time to time up-gradation as new experiments are coming to the surface. Due to the above-mentioned limitation, it is not possible to get a complete gene interaction map, and also, there is a chance of missing out on crucial genes which can act as drug targets.

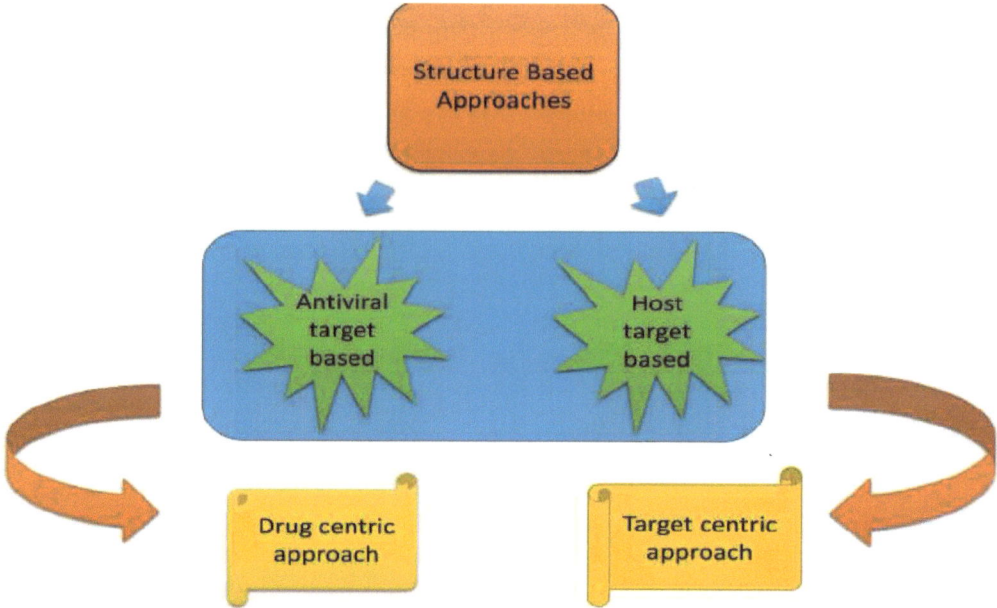

Fig. (5). Diagrammatic presentation of the structure-based approach.

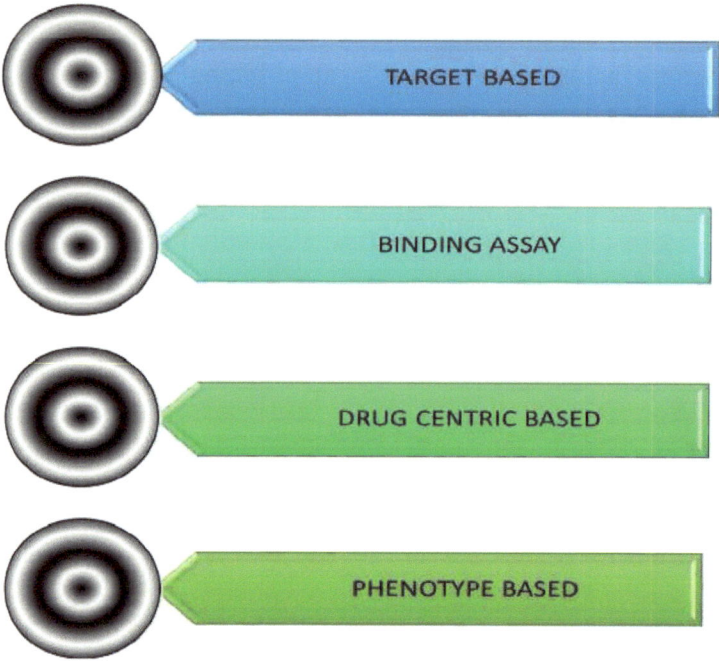

Fig. (6). Types of experimental approaches.

Signature Based

The unique characteristic of a drug is known as the signature of that drug. Its reaction to other drugs and diseases is a unique characteristic of itself. Its chemical structure and biological actions are also unique signatures. For example, in drug-disease interaction, firstly, the gene expression of a cell and tissue can be derived by comparing before and after the treatment. Then the transcriptome signature of the candidate can be obtained after comparison between healthy and diseased conditions. By these changes in the signature profile of the candidate (differentially expressed genes), it can be perfectly scrutinized if it holds any potential against disease treatment. In the drug-drug comparison, two unrelated drugs, both structurally and chemically or pharmacologically having the same mechanism of action, would help us to bring to surface drug target and off-target effects to be investigated for clinical use [50]. CMap (Connectivity Map) is of great help in this regard as it contains millions of profiles for genetic expressions of 5,000 small molecule compounds in the different cell lines. At last, the similarity and dissimilarity in the chemical structure of the drugs should be taken into consideration as they can affect biological activity. The signature-based matching for COVID-19 is successfully applied by Mousavi and their Colleagues [51]. In this, the applied DEG obtained in A549 cells and NHBE (Lung epithelial cell line of humans) in CMap would help them identify any type of similarity between different drug candidates. As a result of it, various drugs-like Lansoprazole, Folic acid, and many other clinically approved drugs, can be used for drug repurposing. This method also has its limitations; there are various unanswered questions like which types of genes are to be selected and how many genes are to be selected for determining the signature of the disease or drugs. Moreover, there is a lack of threshold, which should be adopted while judging a gene expressed differentially when compared with untreated groups. Often a threshold of $\geq$ 1.5 fold change is permissible.

Artificial Intelligence-Based

This approach mainly focuses on various AI models and algorithms, including deep learning architecture and graphical representation learning, which would help in better understanding the massive amount of data on various disease effects obtained from public health surveillance. Though AI-based drug repurposing is at its early stage, it has tremendous potential against COVID-19; twining it with molecular docking to search for potential candidates against COVID-19 can be a handsome and advanced tool. Richardson and Coworkers have utilized a benevolent AI knowledge graph for determining Baricitinib as a potential therapeutic for SARS-CoV-2 [52]. A method has unique challenges associated with it, like the lack of an accurate predictive AI algorithm. The current available

AI tools focus on one data type, which is a crippling soldier against constantly evolving COVID-19. Moreover, such one type of data can give wrong evidence on repurposable drug candidates. Hence, there is a need for evolved AI approach, which should be considered simultaneously multitudinal and multimodal data for accurate production with high precision, and in this regard, MM-RBM (Multimodal Restricted Boltzmann Machine Approach) is believed to be of great help [53].

Experimental Approaches

Following are the types of experimental approaches: -

Target-Based

In this approach, there are a few steps needed to be followed. First is identifying the process followed and the pathway through which disease can progress, followed by target validation to verify how much the target can affect the disease. The second step is determining how the drug and the target interact which is done by using a cell-free binding assay. Then the last step includes identifying the hit and modifying it chemically to increase its efficacy, safety, and stability. For example, Xiu *et al.* found out that spike glycoprotein carries out the fusion between the cells and helps the virus in entering into the host cell. Then, the cell fusion assay has shown the formation of syncytia. So in this regard, peptide, EK-1 and its lipopeptide derivative EK1C4 were used as they have cell fusion inhibition activity and thus reduce syncytia. After that, Vero-6 cells were invaded with live SARS-CoV-2 virus, and the plaque reduction assay was done for proper validation, which was then followed by the Murine model study. Safety measures such as while carrying out cell fusion assay should be in the BSL-2 facility, and while the later validation produces should be under the BSL-3 facility. From the above consideration, it can be concluded that the target-based approach validates lipopeptide EK1C4 to be a potential therapeutic agent for the SARS-CoV-2 virus.

Binding Assay

In this technique, mass spectrometry-based proteomics techniques are used mostly for various pandemics and epidemics. Gordan *et al.* have identified around 332 proteins between coronavirus, and FDA-approved 29 drugs that could be successful in treating COVID-19 is done by using affinity purification mass spectroscopy.

Drug-Centric

In this method, the mechanism of action of an existing drug is utilized in the treatment of other diseases. Various examples can be cited in this field. Thalidomide was previously intended for curing morning sickness in pregnant women but was soon withdrawn from the market due to its potential to cause Phocomelia. But later, it was discovered that the antiangiogenic properties of Thalidomide can be used in multiple myeloma [44]. Another example is valproic acid which was primarily developed to treat the symptoms of bipolar disease and seizures. Later studies found out that it can be used in the treatment of Familial adenomatous polyposis (cancerous growth) due to its effect on histone deacetylase-2. The most famous example nowadays in the pandemic is Remdesivir, whose development is primarily aimed at treating HCV by binding with the viral RdRP resulting in the termination of the RNA chain and inhibiting RNA application of the virus [54]. But studies conducted by Sheahan *et al.* in 2017 showed its potential against the human Corona Virus (SARS-CoV and MERS-CoV) [55]. It has also passed the efficiency test against SARS-CoV-2 conducted by Wang *et al.* Studies have shown that Remdesivir treatment shortens the recovery time for patients suffering from SARS-CoV-2.

Phenotype Based

In this type of screening, observable characteristics or phenotypes play a major role. Cell-based or animal-based models are designed to mimic the disease conditions, and the efficacy of the drug is then checked. The points of consideration are if the disease progression is restricted after the addition of the drug and, if so, what is the mechanism of action. This method of screening has various advantages like there is no restriction or limitations in the mechanism of action, so a variety of drugs can be allowed for testing, and there is no need for identification of a particular drug target or any type of hypothesis on the action of drug towards the diseases. Hence, providing an unbiased opportunity for every candidate. Being easy and readily pursuable various scientists have undertaken this approach like Mok and Colleagues used this method to sort out 121 compounds having anti- SARS-CoV-2 activity, out of which calcitriol has shown inhibiting activity against SARS-CoV-2 in Vero E6 cells. Riva and colleagues have performed large-scale Phenotype screening to find out many entities that positively inhibit the SARS-CoV-2 replication by 40% out of 21 compounds showed dose-dependent inhibition, and 13 compounds are acceptable in therapeutic dose for anti-viral action against SARS-CoV-2. This method also has various limitations associated with it, like it is mostly time-consuming as, for some of the drugs, the mechanism of action is unknown. Moreover, the current pandemic has posed a greater challenge due to its constant evolutionary traits;

along with it, it has multiple pathways for progression, and target identification is not easy in all cases. Around the particle range of 7% to 18% of drugs do not show any proper molecular target. So due to the lack of a definite mechanism of action, the result of serving them as –a hit is fully dependent on their action *in vivo* models. And mimicking the disease conditions and preparing a perfect *in vivo* model is the greatest challenge in this regard.

Drug Repurposing Scenarios In Antiviral Drug Discovery

Same Target – New Virus

If the virus is new and acts on a specific pathway and if the drug existed before for that particular site of action, it could prove to be fruitful. Previously remdesivir being a broad-spectrum anti-viral drug, was being used in MERS and SARS treatment. Studies have shown that it can be used in COVID-19. Similarly, Hydroxychloroquine and chloroquine phosphate were approved to be used in COVID-19.

Same Target New Indication

These types of indications are applied when the drug interacts with the pharmacological targetassociated with a viral infection. Imatinib is an anti-cancer drug that can be used against COVID-19, but originally aimed to inhibit cellular kinase.

New Target New Indications

This pathway is undertaken when the approved drug has new molecular targets, which are an important factor for viral replication. For example- Teicoplanin, itraconazole, and nitazoxanide were able to inhibit virus-infected cells [56].

Animal Models In SARS-CoV-2 Repurposing

Various animal models include Syrian hamsters, mice, and non-human primates for *in-vivo* testing. hACE -2 can serve as a perfect mouse model as it can show SARS-CoV-2 spike glycoprotein interaction with human ACE-2 receptors. It was developed from ICR mice [57]. An experiment is conducted taking 3 groups (wild mice, mock-infected hACE-2 mice, SARS-CoV-2 infected hACE-2 mice). From the studies conducted, it can be concluded that severe weight loss and bristled fur are marked in SARS-CoV-2 infected hACE-2 mice which is absent in other mice types. RT-qPCR results show successful viral loading in the lungs of the hACE-2 mice, and SARS-CoV-2 was obtained from the lungs of the mice, which implies that ACE-2 is an important pathway for the virus to enter the cell. Koch's postulated that SARS-CoV-2 is the causative agent for COVID-19, which can be proved from the above studies conducted. For more severe conditions, K18-hac--2 transgenic mice were used, which was developed in 2006 for SARS-CoV-2. The severe symptoms marked in this type of mouse model include severe disease in the lungs, infection in the brain, pneumonia leading to severe thrombosis, and vasculitis. This mouse model expresses the human ACE-2 receptor under the cytokeratin 18 (K-18) promotor [58]. A rhesus macaque model was suggested by Chandrasekhar and Colleagues to determine the protective immunity building after the primary infection of SARS-CoV-2 [59]. Studies have shown that upon primary infection, viruses can be extracted or marked in both the lower and upper respiratory tract, and less time of recovery is marked along with less viral titer in bronchioalveolar lavage and nasal mucosa. These findings suggest that the body has built up immunity against the virus after the primary infection. This model can also be used to check the efficacy of Remdesivir in SARS-CoV-2 [60]. Treatment with Remdesivir has shown no respiratory disease after the viral infection, less viral titer in the bronchoalveolar lavages is marked, low lung viral load, and less lung tissue damage are marked. The rhesus model was utilized for various vaccine testing as well. Vandoremalen and co-workers utilized this model to check the ChAdOX-1neov-19 vaccine and found that lower viral load and no pneumonia disease are found in macaques [61]. Yu and colleagues also utilized this model for experimenting with the DNA vaccine coding for spike proteins which showed increased humoral and cellular immunity along with significant development in neutralizing antibodies which serves as a protection against SARS-CoV-2 infections. There are various disadvantages also associated with using animal models. First of all, the genetic variability in animal models can lead to variable disease progression in different animals, which may not resemble the viral disease progression in humans due to the lack of ACE2 receptors; wild-type mice were less vulnerable to SARS-CoV-2 infection [57]. Thus, hACE-2 mice are used, but development may be time-consuming, and high cost, and when the next novel pandemic strikes, a better animal model may not be ready. Due to better genetic similarity with primates use of non-human primate models can be better [62]. The limitation is its high cost for housing, caring, and experimentation inaccessibility. As compared to other models, the number of animals available is also less, which can affect the statistical reliability of an experiment.

Limitation of Identified Repurposed Molecules

The main issue with repurposed drugs is finding a perfect dosage that impacts therapeutic efficacy, which is rare for a new drug target interaction. Another limitation in this field is the increased dosage required for obtaining better efficacy, and there is also a need to change the route of administration for the repurposed drug. Safety studies are mandatory when the potency dose of the repurposed drug is beyond the margin. For this reason, achieving a better efficacy and permissible safety dosage is very difficult. So to get a better effect, there is also a need to change the route of drug administration which brings with it various stability issues and other limitations associated with that particular route. Selecting a suitable carrier can be used as a resolution. Various physicochemical properties, release profiles of the repurposed drugs, and Pharmacokinetic, and biodistribution parameters are to be modulated and taken into consideration. As there are no strict regulations for drug repurposing provided by the regulatory bodies or FDA, there is a problem in determining the amount and type of information to be provided to the regulatory bodies in the field of drug repurposing.

Personalized Drug Repurposing

Advances in pharmacogenetics and pharmacogenomics have shown that illness treatment may be significantly better if medicines were given by a person's genomic profile. Genetic, epigenetic, and environmental variables all impact drug responsiveness. The SARS-CoV-2 infection has exhibited a broad range of inter-individual variations, from asymptomatic to severe and deadly illnesses. Another group discovered that chloroquine did not protect the TMPRSS2-positive lung cell line against SARS-CoV-2 infection like Calu-3 [63]. Human genetics may have a role in determining clinical traits and pharmacological reactions, according to one theory. [42, 64] For example, a study of roughly 81 000 genomes and exomes from the normal population found that hydroxychloroquine or chloroquine may only be effective in individuals who are TMPRSS2-deficient and infected with SARS-CoV-2. In the kidney cells of African green monkeys having an absence of TMPRSS2 expression (VeroE6), an international team discovered that hydroxychloroquine exhibits antiviral action, but not in a model of reconstituted human airway epithelium made from primary nasal or bronchial cells. These data obtained underline the relevance of pharmacogenomics research in improving clinical outcomes and medication repurposing success rates. A COVID-19 host genetics program is now ongoing to collect, distribute, and scrutinize data in the quest for genetic groups of COVID-19 susceptibility having severe outcomes, as well as customized therapy. This concept has shown promise in the treatment of a variety of disorders, including cancer [65]. As a result, AI approaches might be used to mine huge amounts of data regarding genetics and genomics to find human genetic variables for SARS-CoV-2 pathogenesis, presenting a new potential for therapeutic repurposing and individualized therapy for Coronavirus patients.

CONCLUSION

During the global pandemic outbreak, finding a better therapeutics option is the need of situation; for this reason, drug repurposing is a boon. Previously known drugs, currently approved and existing FDA drugs can serve as a candidate drug. Drugs that are developed for SARS, MERS, HIV/AIDS, malaria, and anticancer are now being repurposed for the treatment of COVID-19, but the only requirement is their detailed clinical and preclinical studies and their interaction with COVID-19. Additional consideration includes its administration route, dosage, efficacy, and its safety profile. More emphasis should be given to determining and obtaining the clinical and preclinical data along with statistical and *in-silico* analysis. Moreover, the government and pharmaceutical companies must collaborate in loosening the limitation of patent regulations to get better results in drug repurposing. Identifying new therapeutics of old drugs would help in drug development in a shorter time frame, cost-effectiveness, and loss of attrition, thus can serve as a better approach for treatment in corona pandemic.

CONSENT FOR PUBLICATION

Not applicable.

CONFLICT OF INTEREST

The author declares no conflict of interest, financial or otherwise.

ACKNOWLEDGEMENTS

Authors are thankful to the National Institute of Pharmaceutical Education and Research, Raebareli (NIPER-R), Department of Pharmaceuticals, Ministry of Chemicals and Fertilizers, Govt. Of India, for providing support in every possible form. The communication no (NIPER-R/Communication/245) for the submission of this chapter was also provided by the NIPER-R.

REFERENCES

[1]   Hu B, Guo H, Zhou P, Shi ZL. Characteristics of SARS-CoV-2 and COVID-19. Nat Rev Microbiol 2021; 19(3): 141-54.
[http://dx.doi.org/10.1038/s41579-020-00459-7] [PMID: 33024307]

[2]   Usher K, Durkin J, Bhullar N. The COVID-19 pandemic and mental health impacts. Int J Ment Health Nurs 2020; 29(3): 315-8.
[http://dx.doi.org/10.1111/inm.12726] [PMID: 32277578]

[3]   Naqvi AAT, Fatima K, Mohammad T, *et al.* Insights into SARS-CoV-2 genome, structure, evolution, pathogenesis and therapies: Structural genomics approach. Biochim Biophys Acta Mol Basis Dis 2020; 1866(10): 165878.
[http://dx.doi.org/10.1016/j.bbadis.2020.165878] [PMID: 32544429]

[4]   Sahoo BM, Ravi Kumar BVV, Sruti J, Mahapatra MK, Banik BK, Borah P. Drug Repurposing Strategy (DRS): Emerging Approach to Identify Potential Therapeutics for Treatment of Novel Coronavirus Infection. Front Mol Biosci 2021; 8: 628144.
[http://dx.doi.org/10.3389/fmolb.2021.628144] [PMID: 33718434]

[5]   Sultana J, Crisafulli S, Gabbay F, Lynn E, Shakir S, Trifirò G. Challenges for drug repurposing in the COVID-19 pandemic era. Front Pharmacol 2020; 11: 588654.
[http://dx.doi.org/10.3389/fphar.2020.588654] [PMID: 33240091]

[6]   Venkatesan P. Repurposing drugs for treatment of COVID-19. Lancet Respir Med 2021; 9(7): e63.
[http://dx.doi.org/10.1016/S2213-2600(21)00270-8] [PMID: 34090608]

[7]   Singh TU, Parida S, Lingaraju MC, Kesavan M, Kumar D, Singh RK. Drug repurposing approach to fight COVID-19. Pharmacol Rep 2020; 72(6): 1479-508.
[http://dx.doi.org/10.1007/s43440-020-00155-6] [PMID: 32889701]

[8]   Ferner RE, Aronson JK. Remdesivir in covid-19. BMJ 2020; 369: m1610.
[http://dx.doi.org/10.1136/bmj.m1610] [PMID: 32321732]

[9]   Joshi S, Parkar J, Ansari A, *et al.* Role of favipiravir in the treatment of COVID-19. Int J Infect Dis 2021; 102: 501-8.
[http://dx.doi.org/10.1016/j.ijid.2020.10.069] [PMID: 33130203]

[10]   Schoergenhofer C, Jilma B, Stimpfl T, Karolyi M, Zoufaly A. Pharmacokinetics of lopinavir and ritonavir in patients hospitalized with coronavirus disease 2019 (COVID-19). Ann Intern Med 2020; 173(8): 670-2.
[http://dx.doi.org/10.7326/M20-1550] [PMID: 32422065]

[11]   Gasmi A, Peana M, Noor S, *et al.* Chloroquine and hydroxychloroquine in the treatment of COVID-19: the never-ending story. Appl Microbiol Biotechnol 2021; 105(4): 1333-43.
[http://dx.doi.org/10.1007/s00253-021-11094-4] [PMID: 33515285]

[12]   Satarker S, Ahuja T, Banerjee M, *et al.* Hydroxychloroquine in COVID-19: Potential Mechanism of Action Against SARS-CoV-2. Curr Pharmacol Rep 2020; 6(5): 203-11.
[http://dx.doi.org/10.1007/s40495-020-00231-8] [PMID: 32864299]

[13]   Guaraldi G, Meschiari M, Cozzi-Lepri A, *et al.* Tocilizumab in patients with severe COVID-19: a retrospective cohort study. Lancet Rheumatol 2020; 2(8): e474-84.
[http://dx.doi.org/10.1016/S2665-9913(20)30173-9] [PMID: 32835257]

[14]   Chen J, Xia L, Liu L, *et al.* Antiviral Activity and Safety of Darunavir/Cobicistat for the Treatment of COVID-19. Open Forum Infect Dis 2020; 7(7): ofaa241.
[http://dx.doi.org/10.1093/ofid/ofaa241] [PMID: 32671131]

[15]   Khalili JS, Zhu H, Mak NSA, Yan Y, Zhu Y. Novel coronavirus treatment with ribavirin: Groundwork for an evaluation concerning COVID□19. J Med Virol 2020; 92(7): 740-6.
[http://dx.doi.org/10.1002/jmv.25798] [PMID: 32227493]

[16]   Zhu Z, Lu Z, Xu T, *et al.* Arbidol monotherapy is superior to lopinavir/ritonavir in treating COVID-19. J Infect 2020; 81(1): e21-3.
[http://dx.doi.org/10.1016/j.jinf.2020.03.060] [PMID: 32283143]

[17]   Hofmann-Winkler H, Moerer O, Alt-Epping S, *et al.* Camostat mesylate may reduce severity of coronavirus disease 2019 sepsis: a first observation. Crit Care Explor 2020; 2(11): e0284.
[http://dx.doi.org/10.1097/CCE.0000000000000284] [PMID: 33225308]

[18]   Ikeda M, Hayase N, Moriya K, Morimura N. Nafamostat mesylate treatment in combination with favipiravir for patients critically ill with COVID-19: a case series. Crit Care 2020; 24(1): 1-4.
[PMID: 31898531]

[19]   Sayad B, Sobhani M, Khodarahmi R. Sofosbuvir as repurposed antiviral drug against COVID-19: why were we convinced to evaluate the drug in a registered/approved clinical trial? Arch Med Res 2020;

51(6): 577-81.
[http://dx.doi.org/10.1016/j.arcmed.2020.04.018] [PMID: 32387040]

[20]   Nourian A, Khalili H. Sofosbuvir as a potential option for the treatment of COVID-19. Acta Biomed 2020; 91(2): 236-8.
[PMID: 32420958]

[21]   Rogosnitzky M, Okediji P, Koman I. Cepharanthine: a review of the antiviral potential of a Japanese-approved alopecia drug in COVID-19. Pharmacol Rep 2020; 72(6): 1509-16.
[http://dx.doi.org/10.1007/s43440-020-00132-z] [PMID: 32700247]

[22]   Yamamoto N, Yang R, Yoshinaka Y, *et al.* HIV protease inhibitor nelfinavir inhibits replication of SARS-associated coronavirus. Biochem Biophys Res Commun 2004; 318(3): 719-25.
[http://dx.doi.org/10.1016/j.bbrc.2004.04.083] [PMID: 15144898]

[23]   Dechaumes A, Nekoua MP, Belouzard S, *et al.* Fluoxetine can inhibit SARS-CoV-2 *in vitro.* Microorganisms 2021; 9(2): 339-79.
[http://dx.doi.org/10.3390/microorganisms9020339] [PMID: 33572117]

[24]   Schütz D, Ruiz-Blanco YB, Münch J, Kirchhoff F, Sanchez-Garcia E, Müller JA. Peptide and peptide-based inhibitors of SARS-CoV-2 entry. Adv Drug Deliv Rev 2020; 167: 47-65.
[http://dx.doi.org/10.1016/j.addr.2020.11.007] [PMID: 33189768]

[25]   Nhean S, Varela ME, Nguyen YN, *et al.* COVID-19: A Review of Potential Treatments (Corticosteroids, Remdesivir, Tocilizumab, Bamlanivimab/Etesevimab, and Casirivimab/Imdevimab) and Pharmacological Considerations. J Pharm Pract 2021, 1;8971900211048139.
[http://dx.doi.org/10.1177/08971900211048139] [PMID: 34597525]

[26]   Coomes EA, Haghbayan H. Favipiravir, an antiviral for COVID-19? J Antimicrob Chemother 2020; 75(7): 2013-4.
[http://dx.doi.org/10.1093/jac/dkaa171] [PMID: 32417899]

[27]   Hernandez AV, Roman YM, Pasupuleti V, Barboza JJ, White CM. Hydroxychloroquine or chloroquine for treatment or prophylaxis of COVID-19: a living systematic review. Ann Intern Med 2020; 173(4): 287-96.
[http://dx.doi.org/10.7326/M20-2496] [PMID: 32459529]

[28]   Oldfield V, Dhillon S, Plosker GL. Tocilizumab. Drugs 2009; 69(5): 609-32.
[http://dx.doi.org/10.2165/00003495-200969050-00007] [PMID: 19368420]

[29]   McKeage K, Perry CM, Keam SJ. Darunavir. Drugs 2009; 69(4): 477-503.
[http://dx.doi.org/10.2165/00003495-200969040-00007] [PMID: 19323590]

[30]   Glue P. The clinical pharmacology of ribavirin. Semin Liver Dis 1999; 19 (Suppl. 1): 17-24.
[PMID: 10349689]

[31]   Blaising J, Polyak SJ, Pécheur EI. Arbidol as a broad-spectrum antiviral: An update. Antiviral Res 2014; 107: 84-94.
[http://dx.doi.org/10.1016/j.antiviral.2014.04.006] [PMID: 24769245]

[32]   Hoffmann M, Hofmann-Winkler H, Smith JC, *et al.* Camostat mesylate inhibits SARS-CoV-2 activation by TMPRSS2-related proteases and its metabolite GBPA exerts antiviral activity. bioRxiv 2020; 2020.08.05.237651.
[http://dx.doi.org/10.1101/2020.08.05.237651]

[33]   Choi CW, Kang DH, Kim GH, *et al.* Nafamostat mesylate in the prevention of post-ERCP pancreatitis and risk factors for post-ERCP pancreatitis. Gastrointest Endosc 2009; 69(4): e11-8.
[http://dx.doi.org/10.1016/j.gie.2008.10.046] [PMID: 19327467]

[34]   Lawitz E, Mangia A, Wyles D, *et al.* Sofosbuvir for previously untreated chronic hepatitis C infection. N Engl J Med 2013; 368(20): 1878-87.
[http://dx.doi.org/10.1056/NEJMoa1214853] [PMID: 23607594]

[35]   Bailly C. Cepharanthine: An update of its mode of action, pharmacological properties and medical applications. Phytomedicine 2019; 62: 152956.
[http://dx.doi.org/10.1016/j.phymed.2019.152956] [PMID: 31132753]

[36]   Pai VB, Nahata MC. Nelfinavir mesylate: a protease inhibitor. Ann Pharmacother 1999; 33(3): 325-39.
[http://dx.doi.org/10.1345/aph.18089] [PMID: 10200859]

[37]   Khan SA, Al-Balushi K. Combating COVID-19: The role of drug repurposing and medicinal plants. J Infect Public Health 2021; 14(4): 495-503.
[http://dx.doi.org/10.1016/j.jiph.2020.10.012] [PMID: 33743371]

[38]   Beck BR, Shin B, Choi Y, Park S, Kang K. Predicting commercially available antiviral drugs that may act on the novel coronavirus (SARS-CoV-2) through a drug-target interaction deep learning model. Comput Struct Biotechnol J 2020; 18: 784-90.
[http://dx.doi.org/10.1016/j.csbj.2020.03.025] [PMID: 32280433]

[39]   Zeng X, Song X, Ma T, *et al.* Repurpose Open Data to Discover Therapeutics for COVID-19 Using Deep Learning. J Proteome Res 2020; 19(11): 4624-36.
[http://dx.doi.org/10.1021/acs.jproteome.0c00316] [PMID: 32654489]

[40]   Kadioglu O, Saeed M, Greten HJ, Efferth T. Identification of novel compounds against three targets of SARS CoV-2 coronavirus by combined virtual screening and supervised machine learning. Comput Biol Med 2021; 133: 104359.
[http://dx.doi.org/10.1016/j.compbiomed.2021.104359] [PMID: 33845270]

[41]   Hsieh KL, Wang Y, Chen L, *et al.* Drug repurposing for covid-19 using graph neural network with genetic, mechanistic, and epidemiological validation 2020.
[http://dx.doi.org/10.21203/rs.3.rs-114758/v1]

[42]   Ellinghaus D, Degenhardt F. Severe COVID-19 GWAS Group. Genomewide Association Study of Severe COVID-19 with Respiratory Failure. N Engl J Med. 2020; 383(16): 1522-1534.

[43]   Tam V, Patel N, Turcotte M, Bossé Y, Paré G, Meyre D. Benefits and limitations of genome-wide association studies. Nat Rev Genet 2019; 20(8): 467-84.
[http://dx.doi.org/10.1038/s41576-019-0127-1] [PMID: 31068683]

[44]   Ashburn TT, Thor KB. Drug repositioning: identifying and developing new uses for existing drugs. Nat Rev Drug Discov 2004; 3(8): 673-83.
[http://dx.doi.org/10.1038/nrd1468] [PMID: 15286734]

[45]   Zhou Y, Leng X, Mo C, Zou Q, Liu Y, Wang Y. The p53 effector Perp mediates the persistence of $CD4^+$ effector memory T-cell undergoing lymphopenia-induced proliferation. Immunol Lett 2020; 224: 14-20.
[http://dx.doi.org/10.1016/j.imlet.2020.05.001] [PMID: 32473185]

[46]   Lian N, Xie H, Lin S, Huang J, Zhao J, Lin Q. Umifenovir treatment is not associated with improved outcomes in patients with coronavirus disease 2019: a retrospective study. Clin Microbiol Infect 2020; 26(7): 917-21.
[http://dx.doi.org/10.1016/j.cmi.2020.04.026] [PMID: 32344167]

[47]   Elfiky AA. Ribavirin, Remdesivir, Sofosbuvir, Galidesivir, and Tenofovir against SARS-CoV-2 RNA dependent RNA polymerase (RdRp): A molecular docking study. Life Sci 2020; 253: 117592.
[http://dx.doi.org/10.1016/j.lfs.2020.117592] [PMID: 32222463]

[48]   Martin WR, Cheng F. Repurposing of FDA-Approved Toremifene to Treat COVID-19 by Blocking the Spike Glycoprotein and NSP14 of SARS-CoV-2. J Proteome Res 2020; 19(11): 4670-7.
[http://dx.doi.org/10.1021/acs.jproteome.0c00397] [PMID: 32907334]

[49]   Khelfaoui H, Harkati D, Saleh BA. Molecular docking, molecular dynamics simulations and reactivity, studies on approved drugs library targeting ACE2 and SARS-CoV-2 binding with ACE2. J Biomol Struct Dyn 2021; 39(18): 7246-62.

[http://dx.doi.org/10.1080/07391102.2020.1803967] [PMID: 32752951]

[50]   Keiser MJ, Setola V, Irwin JJ, *et al.* Predicting new molecular targets for known drugs. Nature 2009; 462(7270): 175-81.
[http://dx.doi.org/10.1038/nature08506] [PMID: 19881490]

[51]   Mousavi SZ, Rahmanian M, Sami A. A connectivity map-based drug repurposing study and integrative analysis of transcriptomic profiling of SARS-CoV-2 infection. Infect Genet Evol 2020; 86: 104610.
[http://dx.doi.org/10.1016/j.meegid.2020.104610] [PMID: 33130005]

[52]   Richardson P, Griffin I, Tucker C, *et al.* Baricitinib as potential treatment for 2019-nCoV acute respiratory disease. Lancet 2020; 395(10223): e30-1.
[http://dx.doi.org/10.1016/S0140-6736(20)30304-4] [PMID: 32032529]

[53]   Hooshmand SA, Zarei Ghobadi M, Hooshmand SE, Azimzadeh Jamalkandi S, Alavi SM, Masoudi-Nejad A. A multimodal deep learning-based drug repurposing approach for treatment of COVID-19. Mol Divers 2021; 25(3): 1717-30.
[http://dx.doi.org/10.1007/s11030-020-10144-9] [PMID: 32997257]

[54]   Wang M, Cao R, Zhang L, *et al.* Remdesivir and chloroquine effectively inhibit the recently emerged novel coronavirus (2019-nCoV) *in vitro.* Cell Res 2020; 30(3): 269-71.
[http://dx.doi.org/10.1038/s41422-020-0282-0] [PMID: 32020029]

[55]   Sheahan TP, Sims AC, Graham RL, *et al.* Broad-spectrum antiviral GS-5734 inhibits both epidemic and zoonotic coronaviruses. Sci Transl Med 2017; 9(396): eaal3653.
[http://dx.doi.org/10.1126/scitranslmed.aal3653] [PMID: 28659436]

[56]   Ng YL, Salim CK, Chu JJH. Drug repurposing for COVID-19: Approaches, challenges and promising candidates. Pharmacol Ther 2021; 228: 107930.
[http://dx.doi.org/10.1016/j.pharmthera.2021.107930] [PMID: 34174275]

[57]   Bao L, Deng W, Huang B, *et al.* The pathogenicity of SARS-CoV-2 in hACE2 transgenic mice. Nature 2020; 583(7818): 830-3.
[http://dx.doi.org/10.1038/s41586-020-2312-y] [PMID: 32380511]

[58]   Zheng J, Wong LYR, Li K, *et al.* COVID-19 treatments and pathogenesis including anosmia in K18-hACE2 mice. Nature 2021; 589(7843): 603-7.
[http://dx.doi.org/10.1038/s41586-020-2943-z] [PMID: 33166988]

[59]   Chandrashekar A, Liu J, Martinot AJ, *et al.* SARS-CoV-2 infection protects against rechallenge in rhesus macaques. Science 2020; 369(6505): 812-7.
[http://dx.doi.org/10.1126/science.abc4776] [PMID: 32434946]

[60]   Williamson BN, Feldmann F, Schwarz B, *et al.* Clinical benefit of remdesivir in rhesus macaques infected with SARS-CoV-2. Nature 2020; 585(7824): 273-6.
[http://dx.doi.org/10.1038/s41586-020-2423-5] [PMID: 32516797]

[61]   van Doremalen N, Lambe T, Spencer A, *et al.* ChAdOx1 nCoV-19 vaccine prevents SARS-CoV-2 pneumonia in rhesus macaques. Nature 2020; 586(7830): 578-82.
[http://dx.doi.org/10.1038/s41586-020-2608-y] [PMID: 32731258]

[62]   Lu YR, Wang LN, Jin X, *et al.* A preliminary study on the feasibility of gene expression profile of rhesus monkey detected with human microarray. Transplant Proc 2008; 40(2): 598-602.
[http://dx.doi.org/10.1016/j.transproceed.2008.01.029] [PMID: 18374140]

[63]   Hoffmann M, Mösbauer K, Hofmann-Winkler H, *et al.* Chloroquine does not inhibit infection of human lung cells with SARS-CoV-2. Nature 2020; 585(7826): 588-90.
[http://dx.doi.org/10.1038/s41586-020-2575-3] [PMID: 32698190]

[64]   Hou Y, Zhao J, Martin W, *et al.* New insights into genetic susceptibility of COVID-19: an ACE2 and TMPRSS2 polymorphism analysis. BMC Med 2020; 18(1): 216.
[http://dx.doi.org/10.1186/s12916-020-01673-z] [PMID: 32664879]

[65]   Nussinov R, Jang H, Tsai CJ, Cheng F. Review: Precision medicine and driver mutations: Computational methods, functional assays and conformational principles for interpreting cancer drivers. PLOS Comput Biol 2019; 15(3): e1006658.
[http://dx.doi.org/10.1371/journal.pcbi.1006658] [PMID: 30921324]

CHAPTER 5

Repurposed Drugs/Potential Pharmacological Agents Targeting Cytokine Release and Induction of Coagulation in COVID-19

Arpita Singh[1],*, #, Ajay Kumar Verma[2], Anuj Kumar Pandey[2] and Jyoti Bajpai[2]

[1] *Department of Pharmacology, Dr. Ram Manohar Lohia Institute of Medical Sciences, Lucknow, Uttar Pradesh, India,*

[2] *Department of Respiratory Medicine, King George's Medical University, Lucknow, Uttar Pradesh, India*

Abstract: Global public health has been challenged by the coronavirus 2019 (COVID-19) and has been a threat to clinical management to fight this viral infection. Due to the lack of specific therapies, there is a race among the scientific fraternity to find its specific cure to date. COVID-19 symptoms range from mild fatigue to potentially fatal pneumonia, cytokine storm (CS), and multi-organ failure. Hence, investigating the repurposing of current medications for use in the management of COVID-19 patients is a realistic approach. It is prudent to investigate using repurposed medications in the management of COVID-19 patients. In the meantime, researchers are testing a number of antiviral and immunomodulatory medicines to combat the infection. Although antiviral as well as supportive medications are undoubtedly vital in the treatment of COVID-19 patients, anti-inflammatory agents play an essential part in COVID-19 patient care due to their potential to prevent additional injury and organ damage and/or failure. Moreover, COVID-19-mediated infection can be linked with coagulopathy. The most common thrombotic events in COVID-19 are venous thromboembolic (VTE), which are linked with increased severity of disease and poor clinical outcomes. Here, we evaluated medicines that potentially modulate pro-inflammatory cytokines and assist in COVID-19 management. We emphasized various pro-inflammatory cytokines as targets of repurposed drugs and targeted induction coagulation in COVID-19 patients using the available literature and studies.

Keywords: Anticoagulation, Coagulopathy, Cytokine storm, Interleukin-1, Interleukin-6, Pro-inflammatory cytokines, Repurposed drugs, SARS-CoV-2, Thrombosis, Tumor necrosis factor.

---

* **Corresponding author Arpita Singh:** Department of Pharmacology, Dr. Ram Manohar Lohia Institute of Medical Sciences, Lucknow, Uttar Pradesh, India; Tel: +91 9415675163, E-mail: drarpitasingh21@gmail.com
# Authors contributed equally

INTRODUCTION

The coronavirus disease 2019 (COVID-19), caused by the severe acute respiratory syndrome coronavirus-2 (SARS-CoV-2), has posed a significant threat to global public health. It was first reported as some unknown pneumonia cases in Wuhan, Hubei province, China, in December 2019. Still, we are competing with a different and new variant of the coronavirus to survive. This pandemic is one of the most difficult to control crises in the history of the world. The lives of millions of people are threatened, and many more are still fighting this virus lurking in the atmosphere [1, 2]. Due to this unprecedented mortality and morbidity rate, it is the need of the hour to identify potential targets and repurpose drugs as therapeutic options for this disease. Meanwhile, the scientific community is working tirelessly to find a specific cure for this disease. In this critical situation, drug repurposing is not only fast but also a feasible approach to analyse potent medications for fighting this infection with minimal side effects. We should know the structural analysis of drug target proteins and the pathogenesis of SARS- CoV-2 infection to develop therapeutic approaches [3].

Coronaviruses refer to the family Coronaviridae, subfamily *Coronavirinae,* and of the order *Nidovirales,* as per the International Committee on Taxonomy of Viruses. Further, the Coronavirinae subfamily is grouped into 4 genera: *Alphacoronavirus*, *Betacoronavirus*, *Gammacoronavirus,* and *Deltacoronavirus* [4]. SARS-CoV-2 belongs to the betacoronavirus genera (subgenus sarbecovirus). Alpha and Beta Coronaviruses can infect mammals, while Gamma and Delta CoV are able to infect birds [5]. Earlier in the past two decades, two other zoonotic strains of coronaviruses caused severe respiratory illnesses, namely, severe acute respiratory syndrome coronavirus (SARS- CoV) as well as Middle East respiratory syndrome coronavirus (MERS), began to spread globally. In the years 2002 and 2003, SARS- CoV was the cause of severe acute respiratory syndrome (SARS) outbreaks in China, having a mortality rate of 10%, while MERS-CoV emerged in the year 2012, originating from the Arabian peninsula as an epidemic outbreak. The case fatality rate of MERS was much higher (around 35%) than SARS-CoV, while the basic reproductive number of MERS (R_0) was approx 1. It means the infected person can transmit the disease to up to one person [6 - 8].

SARS-CoV-2 is contagious and spreads mostly by respiratory droplets, with a high transmission rate in the first week of infection. The diagnosis of COVID-19 is carried out by a reverse transcription polymerase chain reaction (RT-PCR) test for coronavirus detection. It was observed that people affected by COVID-19 showed a peak viral load in the first week of illness that gradually decreased by the next week. COVID-19 is now known as a disease that can be associated with multi-organ disorders and a broad spectrum of clinical symptoms [6, 8].

Metagenomic RNA sequencing data of the SARS-CoV-2 unveiled 96.2% analogy to bat-CoV Ra TG13 and 79.6% sequence identity to SARS-CoV [9]. Due to this close phylogenetic similarity, bats were supposed to be the natural host of this virus [9].

This chapter briefly discusses the structure, mutation, and pathogenesis of SARS-CoV-2. Moreover, pro-inflammatory cytokines, cytokine storm (CS), COVID-19-associated CS, and pro-inflammatory cytokines as targets of repurposed drugs were presented. Moreover, we have conferred targeting induction of coagulation in COVID-19 patients.

MECHANISM OF PATHOGENESIS IN COVID-19

SARS-CoV-2 Structure and Mutation

SARS-CoV-2 is an enveloped, non-segmented, positive-sense RNA virus [10 - 12]. SARS-CoV-2 is characterised by 4 structural proteins- spike (S), membrane (M), envelope (E), and nucleocapsid (N) proteins, which are primal for infectivity and replication [13 - 17]. There are six functional open reading frames (ORFs) which are arranged in order from 5' to 3': replicase (ORF1a/ORF1b), spike, envelope, membrane, and nucleocapsid [10]. The S protein consists of two subunits-S1 and S2. When S protein bulges from the membrane side, it gives the virus its appearance [18]. The S protein tip has a crowned (Latin corona) structure [18]. Also, the S protein is essential for binding to the angiotensin-converting enzyme 2 (ACE2) receptor, the key point where the virus enters the human body as well as the animal host [19]. In addition, S protein is the main player in immunogenic response and target of vaccines [19, 20]. M protein (~25-30kDa) is a transmembrane protein essential in viral pathogenesis [21]. S2 portion is highly conserved, and it helps in cell membrane fusion [21]. The E protein (8-12 kDa) is poorly understood, but it is supposed that it has a role in viral replication and infectivity [22, 23]. The N protein is involved in viral RNA replication, transcription, and synthesis control [24]. SARS-CoV-2 also features a hemagglutination-esterase (HE) dimer in structure, that binds to sialic acid and reflects esterase activity to aid viral S-protein cell entrance and propagation [25].

Evidence shows that there are unique mutations in the SARS-CoV-2 [26]. SARS-Co-V-2 mutant variants are as follows: UK variant (B.1.1.7), Brazilian variant (P.1) and South African variant (B.1.351) [27, 28]. The main mutation regions (of these variants) are located in spike protein. B.1.1.7 variants are more contagious and spread faster, which may be related to how well they bind to the ACE2 receptor [27, 29].

SARS-CoV-2 Pathogenesis

The infection of SARS-CoV-2 is mediated by the interaction of the viral spike protein with human ACE2 and transmembrane serine protease 2 (TMPRSS2). The receptor-binding domain of S-protein binds to human ACE2's peptidase domain. Virus attachment is started by binding the S protein to the ACE2 receptor. The S-protein is cleaved into S1, which contains the receptor binding site and binds to the peptidase domain of the ACE2 receptor, and S2, which is required for membrane fusion. The cathepsin L pH-dependent cysteine protease alters the structure of the S protein when it interacts with the ACE2 receptor. The viral envelope is then fused to the inner body wall [30]. Other than this, entry depends on the direct TMPRSS2 of the transmembrane protease to activate the ACE2 receptor and S protein, and after this, the viral envelope fuses with the cell membrane of the host, and the nucleocapsid enters the cytoplasm and releases the viral genome [31]. TMPRSS2 is a specific protein in a viral spike protein that activates the viral spike protein by cleaving it at specific sites to gain entry into the cell. SARS-CoV2 uses ACE2 as a receptor for gaining entry into cells.

The viral genome functions as mRNA. And the translation is used to convert two-thirds of the genome constituting (open reading frames) ORF1a and ORF1b into the polyproteins pp1a and pp1ab [32]. The polyproteins and their proteases (PLpro and 3CLpro) are cleaved into 16 non-structural proteins to form a replicase-transcriptase complex (RTC) [32]. RTC's main protein is RNA-dependent RNA polymerase (RdRp), which arbitrates sense mRNA to synthesise negative sense subgenomic RNA, which is then transcribed into sense mRNA and positive mRNA replicates in the viral particle's genome [32]. And the rest of the genome following ORF is translated into the structural proteins S, E, M, and N in the endoplasmic reticulum (ER). Further, structural proteins move to the golgi apparatus, and there M protein directs protein-protein interaction, which is used for the assembly of proteins to form viral particles. Secretory vesicles are used to transfer viral particles through exocytosis for release [32].

The peak viral load of COVID-19 patients appears in the 1st week of onset and then decreases gradually in the second week. That explains why SARS-CoV-2 is contagious and exhibits high infectivity in the 1st week of infection. Studies have found that the severity of symptoms is related to age. Elderly people show more severe symptoms because of lowered immunity and due to associated co-morbidities like cardiovascular disease, diabetes, lung disease, cancer, *etc.* that influence their collective immunity as well as higher expression of ACE2 receptors [33, 34].

VARIOUS PRO-INFLAMMATORY CYTOKINES AS TARGET OF REPURPOSED DRUGS

Cytokines, Types and Cytokine Storm

Cytokines

Cytokines are small proteins secreted by cells that specifically influence cell contacts and communication [35]. Lymphokines (produced by lymphocytes), monokines (produced by monocytes), chemokines (having chemotactic action), and interleukin (produced by one leukocyte and acting on the other leukocytes) are some of the major names for cytokines [35]. In some cases, cytokines can act on the cells that produce them (autocrine action), nearby cells (paracrine action), and distant cells (endocrine action) [35]. Pleiotropy occurs when Cytokine and/or a single cytokine act on multiple cell types. The activity of cytokines is redundant, which means that different cytokines can trigger comparable processes. They are frequently made in a cascade, with one cytokine promoting the synthesis of others by its target cells. Cytokines can work together (synergistic) or against each other (antagonistic).

Types of Cytokines

Regulatory cytokines that promote inflammation are referred to as pro-inflammatory cytokines. Additionally, the balance of pro-inflammatory and anti-inflammatory cytokines regulates the outcome of an inflammatory response. Additionally, activated macrophages create pro-inflammatory cytokines that play a role in the activation of inflammatory processes. Interleukin (IL)-1 and tumour necrosis factor (TNF) are primary pro-inflammatory cytokines that cause fever, tissue destruction, inflammation, and even shock and death in some cases when given to humans. Endothelium adhesion molecules are activated by IL-1 and TNF and are essential for leukocyte attachment to the endothelial surface just before emigration into tissues. Furthermore, IL-1 and TNF work together in this process. Inflammation by pro-inflammatory cytokines is evolved by a group of gene products which are rarely produced in healthy people. Although it is induced by inflammatory products such as endotoxins, the pro-inflammatory cytokines IL-1 and TNF (and, in some cases, IFN-γ) effectively increase the expression of linked genes. IL-1 and TNF are inflammatory mediators that target the endothelium and are triggered by infections, ischemia, trauma, immune-activated T cells, and/or toxins. In addition, IL-1 and TNF collaborate in this process. The primary pro-inflammatory cytokines that play a significant role in the early reactions are IL1-, IL1, IL6, and TNF-. of the IL20 family, IFN-γ, IL33, LIF, CNTF, GM-CSF, OSM, TGF-beta, IL-11, IL-12, IL-17, IL-18, IL-8, and other chemokines that attract inflammatory cells are among the additional pro-inflammatory mediators. Endogenous pyrogens such as IL-1, IL-6, and TNF-α stimulate the production of pro-inflammatory cytokines and secondary mediators by macrophages and mesenchymal cells, resulting in the release of inflammatory cells or acute phase proteins. There is a lot of evidence that pro-inflammatory cytokines like IL-1, IL-6, and TNF-alpha are engaged in the pathological pain process.

Anti-inflammatory cytokines, a class of immunoregulatory molecules, regulate pro-inflammatory cytokines. Anti-inflammatory cytokines such as interleukin (IL)-1 receptor antagonist, IL-4, IL-10, IL-11, and IL-13 are all crucial. Depending on the situation, leukaemia inhibitory factor, interferon, IL-6, and transforming growth factor (TGF) are classified as either anti-inflammatory or pro-inflammatory cytokines.

Cytokine Storm (CS)

Although an uncontrolled, cytokine-mediated response was first described in the 1980s in the context of malaria and sepsis [36, 37] and later in the 2000s in pancreatitis [38], variola virus [39], and influenza virus H5N1 [40]. The term cytokine storm (CS) was first introduced in the year 1993 in the context of graft vs. host disease. CS can be caused directly by different types of pathogens as well as certain medicines [41]. It is also termed an "infusion reaction" or "cytokine release syndrome." Adoptive T-cell therapies [42], monoclonal antibody regimens [43, 44], and immune checkpoint blockade inhibitors [45 - 47] are all known to cause CS. A stressed or infected cell activates a vast number of WBC, B-cells, T-cells, natural killer (NK) cells, dendritic cells, macrophages, and monocytes, *via* receptor-ligand interactions [41]. In a positive feedback loop, inflammatory cytokines are released through activating additional WBCs. CS is initiated locally after an infection spreads to the rest of the body *via* systemic circulation. Heat, pain, redness, swelling, and loss of function, among other things, are all classical signs of inflammation [41]. The localised response includes protective mechanisms such as increased blood circulation, facilitation of leucocyte extravasation as well as delivery of plasma proteins to the site of injury, an increase in body temperature (beneficial in cases of bacterial infection), and pain triggering [41].

COVID-19-associated Cytokine Storm

COVID-19 symptoms range from mild fatigue to potentially fatal pneumonia, cytokine storm, and multi-organ failure. CS has also been documented in SARS patients, and it has been linked to poor outcomes [48]. However, the mechanisms of COVID-19 lung injury & multi-organ failure remain unclear. The results of hemophagocytosis & increased cytokine levels, and the beneficial effects of immunosuppressive agents in the patients (especially the ill), suggest that CS may play an important role in COVID-19 pathogenesis [49 - 51]. In patients with COVID-19–associated CS, IL-1, IL-6, IP-10, TNF, interferon-γ, macrophage inflammatory protein (MIP)-1, and VEGF levels are elevated [52, 53]. High levels of IL-6 are closely linked to a shorter life expectancy [54]. COVID-19 increases the frequency of activated CD4+, CD8+, and T-cells in the blood, as well as plasmablasts [55]. Aside from increased systemic cytokines and activated immune cells, COVID-19 patients have had a number of clinical and biochemical abnormalities, including increased levels of CRP and d-dimer, hypoalbuminemia, and renal dysfunction. All of these are shown in CS syndrome [56].

The exact function of the CS has yet to be elucidated. However, it tends to be associated with the severity of ARDS in COVID-19, and it is evident that cytokine balance may be a meaningful clinical assessment in the patient's therapy. Three distinct clinical phenotypes have been defined based on the production of cytokines mediated by SARS-CoV-2 immunological activation: a) mild – characterised by cytokine drizzle; b) severe – characterised by a storm; c) critical – characterised by cytokine "hurricane" [57]. Furthermore, establishing an effective treatment requires understanding the mechanism, as this disease evolves from mild to severe as a result of immunological dysfunction and cytokine dysregulation [58].

SARS-CoV-2 infection induces a down-regulation of the ACE2 protein, which contributes to the higher production of vasoconstrictor Ang II. The AngII-AT1R axis activates nuclear factor B (NFB) signalling and metalloprotease 17 (ADAM17), which leads to the synthesis of mature epidermal growth factor receptor (EGFR) ligands and TNF-α [24]. The activation of NFB and STAT3 results in a state of hyperinflammation [59]. Additionally, the viral infection activates macrophages, neutrophils, and NK cells, all of which produce pro-inflammatory cytokines. IFN, INF, IL-1, IL-2, TNF, IL-6, and other cytokines are the initial line of defence against pathogens. For example, toll-like receptors (TLRs) are recognised by pathogen-associated molecular patterns (PAMPs) [60]. TLR activation induces the release of inflammatory cytokines, *e.g.*, IL-6, TNF, and IL-1 [61]. Then, in a mild phenotype, adaptive immune cells contribute to the enhancement of the immunological response by directly attacking virus-infected cells or by releasing various pro-inflammatory cytokines [60].

The CS syndrome may arise in severe COVID-19 individuals. Due to cell lysis, this mechanism tends to release an excess amount of pro-inflammatory cytokines [62]. Macrophages (active) contribute by increasing the production of IL-6, IL-1, IL-8, IL-18, granulocyte-macrophage colony-stimulating factor (GMCSF), chemokine CX-C motif ligand (CXCL)-9, and CXCL-10 [62, 63]. Because of the increased vascular permeability caused by a virus infection, a massive amount of blood and fluid enters the alveoli, causing serious damage to the host cells and respiratory failure [64, 65]. The upregulation of T-cells and production of PICs, including IL-6, are related to SARS-CoV-2-induced pneumonia [66]. COVID-19 pulmonary immunopathology is defined by a number of characteristics, but the cytokine profile shows an increase in IL-1, IL-2, IL-6, IL-17, IL-8, TNF, and CCL-2 [67]. IL-6 is important in aggravating the patient's respiratory status and also the COVID-19 severity [66]. IL-6 plays a major role in lung repair responses during viral (SARS-CoV-2) infections by inducing the development of acute phase proteins like CRP-proteins [68].

Pro-inflammatory Cytokines

Interleukins

Pro-inflammatory cytokines are listed in Table **1**. Interleukins (ILs) are proteins that mediate pro- and anti-inflammatory responses, as well as immune cell development and activation, considered to be engaged only in leucocyte-to-leucocyte communication (thus named interleukin); it is now recognised as being produced by different cell types. IL-1 stimulates IL-2 secretion, which is essential for T-cell homeostasis [69], as well as IL-2 receptor expression [70, 71]. IL-1 increases acute-phase signaling, immune cell trafficking at the primary site of infection, secondary cytokine production, and epithelial cell activation. The acute phase response to infection is characterised by a number of pro-inflammatory effects (local and systemic), including a rise in specific cytokine production related to viral clearance. IL-1 has a costimulatory function only on TH2 cells, with hardly any impact on TH1 cells [71]. The IL-1RI high-affinity receptor is mainly expressed on TH2 cells [72]. In hypersensitivity models *viz.* IL-1, mice had fewer IL-4 and IL-5 levels when compared with the control group, reducing allergy symptoms [73].

Table 1. Pro-inflammatory cytokines and growth factors with their main cell sources and function.

S.No.	Pro-inflammatory Cytokines and Growth Factors	Chief Cell Sources	Function
1.	Interleukin-1(IL-1)	Macrophages, epithelial cells; pyroptotic cells	Pyrogenic activity, macrophage activation, and Th17 cell activation
2.	Interleukin-6 (IL-6)	Macrophages, T cells, endothelial cells	Increased antibody production, pyrogenic function, and stimulation of acute-phase reactants
3.	Interleukin-18 (IL-18)	Monocytes, macrophages, dendritic cells	Activation of the Th1 pathway, which works in conjunction with interleukin-12.

(Table 1) cont.....

S.No.	Pro-inflammatory Cytokines and Growth Factors	Chief Cell Sources	Function
4.	Interleukin-33(IL-33)	Macrophages, dendritic cells, mast cells, epithelial cells	Th1 and Th2 cell amplification, as well as activation of NK cells, CTLs, and mast cells
5.	Interferon-γ (IFN- γ)	Th1 cells, CTLs, group 1 innate lymphoid cells, and NK cells	Activation of macrophages
6.	Tumor necrosis factor (TNF)	Macrophages, T cells, NK cells, mast cells	Induction of fever and enhancement of systemic inflammation; increasing vascular permeability; and pyrogenic function
7.	Granulocyte-macrophage colony-stimulating factor (GM-CSF)	Th17 cells, macrophages, mast cells, NK cells	Myeloid cell activation and migration to inflammatory sites

IL-10 stimulates in the same way that IL-2 and IL-7 do. Antigen-presenting cells (APC), which are associated with the development and activation of CD8 T cells and TH cells, are hypothesised to secrete IL-10 as a feedback reaction to elevated levels of IFN-and IL-6. In the instance of COVID-19, it seems that IL-10, a powerful immunological modulator, is considered a key indicator of immune disorder. Increased IL-10 levels are not related to the immunological disadvantage, but they do point to the latent immune response to regulate the CS [74], which appears to be too late. In a late regulatory attempt by the immune system, IL-4, a TH2 cytokine and an inflammatory suppressor, rises in ICU patients [52]. ILs, unlike IFNs, are not the prototypical antiviral cytokines, but they do have an impact on cytokine storm morbidity.

IL-6 is a major player in inflammation and the COVID-19 pandemic. IL-6 influences the activity of different cell types. As a result, it is referred to as a pleiotropic cytokine because it functions as both a pro-inflammatory cytokine as well as an anti-inflammatory myokine (muscle cells produce this type of cytokine in response to muscular contraction). An IL6/IL6R complex is formed when IL-6 is produced and binds to its soluble receptor. IL-6 binds to a receptor, which is found on a wide range of immune cells. The IL-6 receptor-signalling complex is made up of 2 transmembrane IL-6 binding chains, 2 soluble IL-6 receptors, and 2 cytoplasmic signalling molecules. The cytoplasmic signalling molecule IL-6 is shared by IL-6 members, including leukaemia inhibitory factors, IL-22, IL-25, and IL-27. In the central nervous system, IL-6 stimulates the development of CD4 T cells (naive) into effector and helper cells [75]. By linking innate immunity to adaptive immunological responses, IL-6 promotes TH7 differentiation [76], and the activation and differentiation of cytotoxic CD8T cells [77]. Furthermore, IL-6 inhibits T regulatory T CD4+, CD25+, and FOXP3 cells, which contributes to the development of autoimmune disorders [78]. In addition to IL-21, IL-6 affects immunoglobulin synthesis indirectly by boosting T-follicular helper cell, plasma cell, and B cell development. Aside from that, some viruses have the ability to alter the intracellular activities that lead to inflammation as well as the release of IL-6.

Interleukin-18 belongs to the IL-1 family [79], which has been linked to CS. Inflammasomes activate interleukin-18 and interleukin-1 from precursors. The inflammasome is a sterile stressor cytosolic sensor that detects pathogenic microorganisms and activates caspase-1 during pyroptosis, causing the inactive precursor of IL-1 and IL-18 to become active forms [80, 81]. The chief sources of bioactive IL-18, which has numerous pro-inflammatory effects, are macrophages and dendritic cells. Most importantly, it stimulates interferon-secretion from T and NK cells, promoting Th1-type inflammatory responses when combined with IL-12 or IL-15.The IL-18 receptor is expressed constitutively on NK cells and is activated on the majority of T cells. IL-1 and IL-18 are also powerful inducers of macrophage IL-6 secretion [82]. Interleukin-18's pro-inflammatory effects are normally suppressed by the IL-18–binding protein (IL18BP), which prevents IL-18 from binding to respective receptors [83]. The ratio of free IL-18 to bound IL-18B in serum is a primary predictor of the severity of macrophage activation syndrome [84, 85]. Tadekinig, a recombinant IL18BP, is being studied as a treatment for hyperinflammation.

IL-6 levels are a reliable predictor of the severity of the disease and ventilation support in the SARS-CoV-2 outbreak [86 - 88]. In COVID-19, a CT scan of the lung of a patient with vast bilateral lobular pneumonia is related to higher levels of IL-1, IL-7, IL-8, and IL-9 in the initial plasma concentration [52]. These cytokines are supposed to be released by injured cells and are early immune factors of the COVID-19 immune response. Surprisingly, this increment was similar in ICU as well as non-ICU patients, implying a significant role in COVID-19 immunopathology [52]. Furthermore, IL-2 and IL-7 levels were higher in ICU patients than in non-ICU patients [52, 89]. Pedersen *et al.* discussed how elevated levels of IL-6 in the presence of TNF-α and IL-10 are strongly associated with a lower chance of recovery and the need for ICU admission [74]. Furthermore, mild to moderate IL-6 levels were found to correlate with moderate to severe cases. Prompetchara *et al.* demonstrated that there was a 52% increase in IL-6 levels in ICU patients in comparison to non-ICU patients [90].

Transforming Growth Factor (TNF)

Interferons (IFN)

Interferons (IFN) are primal cytokines allied in innate immunity to bacteria as well as viruses. Type-I & Type-III IFN are generated by all nucleated cells after viral infection; IFN-α is primarily produced by leucocytes, and IFN-β by fibroblasts. Type-II IFN (IFN-γ) is produced by macrophages and natural killer (NK) cells in response to viral and/or intracellular bacterial infections. Additionally, during antigen-specific immunity, IFN-γ is also secreted by T helper (TH) CD4 [95] as well as CD8 cytotoxic T lymphocyte (CTL) effector T cells [96]. After cognate receptor binding (IFNAR1/IFNAR2 for Type I interferons, IFN-R1/IFN-R2 for Type-II IFN, receptor complex IL-28R/IL -10R for Type III— lambda IFN), IFN activates a heterogeneous network of downstream signalling, resulting in transcription factor activation and induction of a variety of IFN-γ stimulated genes with antiviral, immunomodulatory, and anti-proliferative properties.

IFN-γ levels in COVID-19 increased in parallel to viral load [52]. Delayed peak, which coincided with a reduction in lymphocyte counts, resulted in greater neutrophil infiltration of the lungs' alveoli and worsening of the disease condition [52, 74, 97]. IFN-γ has previously been linked to disease severity. Elevated levels of IFN-γ were related to not only pulmonary inflammation but also lung damage in SARS-CoV-1 and MERS-CoV [98, 99]; both were classical signs of worsening. The combination of IFN- γ and IL -6 has been demonstrated to better predict COVID-19 patients decline and ICU admission [41, 74, 97]. IFN-γ has been recognized as CD4 T cells, which are source of IFN-γ, that helps to promote CD8 T cell differentiation and activate cytotoxic capacity. CD4 TH cells secrete granulocyte and monocyte colony-stimulating factors, which promotes monocyte differentiation (CD16+ CD14+ CD45+) and is a source of IFN- γ in the blood.

Granulocyte-Macrophage Colony-Stimulating Factor (GM-CSF)

GM-CSF is a myelopoietic growth factor and pro-inflammatory cytokine that is essential for alveolar macrophage homeostasis, in different immune diseases and lung inflammation [100]. In COVID- 19 clinical trials, both GM-CSF administration and inhibition are being tested for therapeutic purposes. Macrophage colony-stimulating factor (M-CSF), granulocyte colony-stimulating factor (G-CSF), and GM-CSF are all involved in myelopoiesis, which is the process of production of monocytes, macrophages, dendritic cells, and granulocytes by progenitor cells. Importantly, GM- CSF is identified as a crucial homeostatic factor in lung alveoli, where it is formed at low levels to promote the development and long-term survival of alveolar macrophages [101, 102]. Thus, GM-CSF plays a vital role in lung health and may be essential for host defence. GM-CSF is a critical cytokine that can manage not only innate but also adaptive immune responses and can be produced by a variety of cell types, *e.g.*, epithelial cells and leukocytes. GM-CSF has two major functions in the immune response: it polarises mature myeloid cells into pro-inflammatory phenotypes (paracrine/autocrine function), and it regulates emergency myelopoiesis, expanding and mobilising progenitor myeloid cells to sites of inflammation (endocrine function) [103]. It has been postulated that GM CSF acts as the primary communication link between inflammatory lymphoid and myeloid cells [104].

In the COVID-19 context, different therapeutic strategies will occur in a short span of time (≤ 2 weeks), reducing the lung toxicity risk. Besides that, mAb administration timing could be critical. However, in the early stages of the disease, GM-CSF may be beneficial in sustaining alveolar macrophages and functions at viral assault, whereas in the later stages of the disease, reducing GM-CSF may be capable of lowering the underlying pathology of the CS and myeloid cell-induced lung damage [105].

Drugs Repurposing

Drug repositioning, reprofiling, repurposing, or retasking is the process of looking at current drugs to find new ways to use them [106]. A repurposed drug (either in development or approved) already has a proven safety as well as toxicity profile as per Phase I or Phase II successful clinical trials. When compared to bringing a new drug to market, the cost of launching a repurposed drug to market is expected to be much cheaper. Despite the fact that the clinical phase III and other aspects of developing a new drug are similar, repurposing has several advantages over developing a new drug from the ground up, including reduced developmental time and costs, a lesser chance of failure, and better pharmaceutical support from the production and supply to the patients who require treatment the most urgently [107].

There are numerous targets for drug repurposing. However, here we will focus on pro-inflammatory cytokines as a target of repurposed drugs. To date, different classes of medicines are being proposed to minimise the COVID-19 risk. Some of these medications, *viz.* chloroquine (CQ), and hydroxychloroquine (HCQ), have produced an unjustifiable craze due to indiscriminate use as prophylaxis in many countries, such as Brazil and the USA [108]. Though, not the major aim of many medications now employed in the management of COVID-19, there is mounting evidence that the CS may have a considerable effect on the development of the illness, particularly in seriously ill patients [58]. Albeit, there is a paucity of evidence about how these treatments might help to direct key cytokines and help towards the recovery of patients. Several medications which have been examined for their utility in COVID-19 possess anti-inflammatory properties in various diseases and are being explored against the hyperinflammation generated by

SAR-CoV-2 infection. Understanding the molecular targets of these medications in SAR-CoV-2 infection, and the impact on immunological responses, can assist in pitching the route for empirical techniques. Antiviral, anti-inflammatory, antineoplastic, anti-rheumatic, and antiparasitic drugs are some of the pharmacological classes indicated for use in COVID-19 care that may influence the inflammatory process. These medications have been demonstrated to have beneficial effects on COVID-19 patients.

Repurposed Drugs Targeting Pro-inflammatory Cytokines

Several recent investigations have discovered interesting therapeutic candidates that, by blocking various components of COVID-19, may be beneficial against COVID-19. These include antiviral drugs [atazanavir, favipiravir, IFN- 2b (interferon), remdesivir, lopinavir-ritonavir, ribavirin, and umifenovir], anti-rheumatic drugs (anakinara, baricitinib, etanerecpt, infliximab, tocilizumab), anti-inflammatory drugs (indomethacin, thalidomide, corticosteroids), antineoplastic drugs (ibrutinib, ruxolitinib), antibiotics (azithromycin), antiparasitic drugs (chloroquine, hydroxychloroquine, ivermectin, nitazoxanide), monoclonal antibodies (otilimab, gimsilumab, lenzilumab, TJM2, mavrilimumab, namilumab), and other colchicines, sargramostim, *etc.* (Table **2**) [109]. Reports of *in silico*, preclinical, and clinical investigations have indicated that these medicines could improve clinically in SARS-CoV-2 infected patients by lowering virus load as well as minimising the CS.

Table 2. Different drugs and cytokines involved in management of COVID-19.

S.No.	Drug	Mechanism in Management of COVID-19	Cytokines
1	Remdesivir	RNA polymerase inhibitor	$\downarrow$TNF-α, $\downarrow$IL-1β $\downarrow$IL-6, $\downarrow$IL-18
2	Umifenovir	The trimerization of spike glycoprotein of SARS-CoV-2 is blocked	$\downarrow$TNF-α,$\downarrow$IL-6 $\downarrow$IL-8, $\downarrow$IL-10
3	Favipiravir	Interferes with viral replication	$\downarrow$ TNF-α
4	IFN-α2b (interferon)	Inhibits the replication of both SARS-CoV and MERS-CoV	$\uparrow$IL-10 $\uparrow$IL-2, TNF-α
5	Tocilizumab	Anti-IL6R recombinant monoclonal antibody binds to both soluble and membrane-bound IL6R to block IL6-mediated signalling.	$\uparrow$**IL-6, Inhibiting IL-6 Signal transduction**
6	Anakinara	IL-1 receptor antagonist	$\downarrow$TNF-α, $\downarrow$ IL-1β, $\downarrow$ IL-6
7	Baricitinib	Disrupts the transit and intracellular assembly of SARS-CoV-2 into target cells by interfering with AAK1. And by inhibiting clathrin-mediated endocytosis, prevents viral infection of cells.	$\downarrow$TNF-α, $\downarrow$ IL-4, $\downarrow$ IL-6

(Table 2) cont.....

S.No.	Drug	Mechanism in Management of COVID-19	Cytokines
8	Infliximab	TNF-α inhibitor	↓TNF-α, ↓IL-1, ↓IL-6, ↓IL-8
9	Indomethacin	Inhibition of viral replication and infectious viral particle production.	↓TNF-α, ↓IL-1β, ↓IL-6, ↓IL-8
10	Corticosteroids	Inhibits the NFκB transcription factor.	↓TNF-α, ↓IL-1, ↓IL-2, ↓IL-3, ↓IL-5, ↓IL-6, ↓IL-8, ↑IL-10, ↑IL-12, ↓IL-13, ↓IL-15, ↓IFN-β, ↓IFN-λ1, ↓IFN-γ
11	Enalapril	Reduces the interaction between viral protein and ACE2, affecting the internalization of the virus	↓TNF-α, ↓IL-1β, ↑IL-2, ↓IL-6, ↓IL-8, ↑IL-10, ↓IL-12
12	Losartan	Reduces the interaction between viral protein and ACE2	↓TNF-α, ↓IL-1β, ↓IL-6
13	Telmisartan	Reduces the interaction between viral protein and ACE2	↓TNF-α, ↓IL-1β, ↓IL-6, ↓IL-8, ↑IL-10
14	Ibrutinib	Prevents both B-cell activation and B-cell mediated signaling	↓TNF-α, ↓IL-6, ↓IL-8, ↓IL-10
15	Ruxolitinib	Janus kinase inhibitors	↓TNF-α, ↓IL-6
16	Azithromycin	Binds to the 50S ribosomal subunit, affects bacterial protein synthesis	↓TNF-α, ↓IL-6, ↓L-8, ↑IL-10
17	Chloroquine	Alters the pH in the lysosomes, prevents viral fusion and replication, spike (S)-protein angiotensin converting enzyme 2 (ACE2) blockers	↓TNF-α, ↓IL-6, ↓IL-18
18	Hydroxychloroquine	Inhibition of the SARS-CoV cellular receptor (ACE2), viral membrane fusion in the host, nucleic acid replication, new virus transport, and virus release.	↓TNF-α, ↑IL-4, ↓IL-6, ↑IL-10, ↓IL-18, ↓IFN-γ
19	Ivermectin	Inhibition of nuclear transport activity	↓TNF-α, ↓IL-1ss, ↓IL-4, ↓IL-5, ↓IL-6, ↓IL-13
20	Nitazoxanide	Affect the production of viral genomes, prevents viral entrance and inhibits N-glycosylation.	↓TNF-α, ↓IL-1β, ↓IL-6

(Table 2) cont.....

S.No.	Drug	Mechanism in Management of COVID-19	Cytokines
21	Colchicine	Non-selective NLRP3 inflammasome inhibitor, anti-inflammatory actions	↓TNF-α, ↓IL-1β ↓IL 6, ↓IL-18

IL, Interleukin; IFNs, Interferons; TNF, Tumor necrosis factor; MERS-CoV, Middle East Respiratory Syndrome Coronavirus; SARS-CoV-2, Severe Acute Respiratory Syndrome Coronavirus 2; AAK1, AP2-associated protein kinase; IL6R, IL-6 receptor; ACE2: Angiotensin-converting enzyme 2; ACEIs, Angiotensin-converting enzyme inhibitors; ARBs: Angiotensin II type 1 receptor blockers; NLRP3, NOD-, LRR- and pyrin domain-containing protein 3.

As shown in Table **2**, the primary action of antiviral medications in the treatment of COVID-19 is to tamper with viral replication or block fusion in the membrane [110]. However, reducing viral load is one of the modes of action of antiviral medicines. For example, antiviral drugs like atazanavir, remdesivir, favipiravir, umifenovir, and lopinavir-ritonavir have been shown in studies to have antiviral properties indirectly, and also show anti- inflammatory properties as their ability to modulate the inflammatory mediators' production [109 - 115]. According to other research, the COVID- 19 severity may be determined by the extent of the CS, and medications that just reduce viremia may be ineffective at this point [52, 116]. Hence, antiviral medications with anti-inflammatory action may be useful in the management of COVID-19 because of their ability to reduce cellular damage induced by the hyper-inflammatory process, thereby reducing the severity of the infection.

Rheumatological drugs are also being investigated in respect of SARS-CoV-2. The application of anti-rheumatic and anti-inflammatory medicines is justified by the CS which occurs in COVID-19 [117], particularly in poor prognosis and T-cell depleted patients [52]. Controlling CS is critical in the prevention of SARS-CoV-2 infection. Several anti-rheumatic medicines' principal mechanisms of action are on the suppression of inflammatory cascades, such as inhibiting TNF-α, IL- 1Ra, IL-6 receptors, and working as Janus kinase (JAK) inhibitors [118 - 121]. It is clear that the role of IL-6 in COVID-19 pathology, neutralisation of IL-6/IL-6r *via* tocilizumab (a monoclonal antibody, recombinant humanised anti-IL-6r), sarilumab (a recombinant humanised anti-IL6r), and siltuximab (a recombinant human-mouse chimeric monoclonal antibody that binds IL-6) may attenuate CS and also impede renal function impairment [122 - 124]. Anakinra, a drug that blocks IL-1, is another therapeutic option. Anakinra is used to block the pathological effects of IL-1α and IL-1β receptors. Two different cohort studies [125, 126] looked at the clinical effectiveness and found it to be promising. In the absence of randomised trials, the FDA advises health professionals to proceed with caution [127]. Infliximab, a TNF-α inhibitor used to treat Crohn's disease, has been shown to have the capacity to influence the CS associated with COVID-19. The drop in cytokine concentrations caused by infliximab treatment could be linked to p38MAPK pathway downregulation [128].

Due to their ability to reduce the release of inflammatory mediators like IL-6, TNF-α, and IL-1, anti-inflammatory medications have been proposed as adjuvant medicines to reduce the COVID-19 adverse condition [129]. Non-steroidal anti-inflammatory medicines have been shown in studies to be promising possibilities for the treatment of COVID-19. Out of them, indomethacin, which is a non-selective cyclooxygenase inhibitor, has attracted because of its effective *in-vitro* antiviral activity against human SARS-CoV-1 and human SARS-CoV-2 at lesser concentrations [130, 131]. Indomethacin's antiviral action has been linked to viral replication inhibition [132]. Although, another intriguing pharmacological action of this drug is that it could aid COVID-19 patient recovery as its ability to control cytokine production (decreases the release of IL-6) [129, 133, 134]. Indomethacin's potential to reduce inflammatory processes, combined with its antiviral capabilities, makes it a promising contender against COVID-19. Although, scientific trials have not been conducted to evaluate the efficacy of indomethacin for COVID-19, corticosteroids have greater immune activation that may alleviate the systemic inflammatory responses seen in ARDS by lowering the CS. Currently, the use of systemic corticosteroids in COVID-19 is restricted to patients with potentially fatal symptoms related to the CS as well as those with increased serum D-Dimer levels [135]. Thalidomide, another medication, can decrease neutrophil chemotaxis at the inflammation site, limit the production of reactive oxygen species (ROS), and also modify the inflammatory process [136].

Enalapril, an angiotensin-converting-enzyme inhibitor (ACEi), increased IL-10 and IL- 2 levels [137], and decreased TNF-α, IL-1, IL-6, IL -8, and IL-12 production [138, 139], while telmisartan, an AT1R antagonist, decreased TNFα-, IL-1, IL-6, and IL -8 levels [140, 141], confirms the anti-inflammatory function of ACEI/Losartan, an angiotensin II receptor antagonist with few adverse effects, is similarly thought to be protective against COVID-19 infection [142]. Losartan, for instance, has been demonstrated to increase ACE2 expression *in vivo* [143], hence avoiding coronavirus superinfections [142]. Furthermore, losartan 21 alleviates COVID-19 symptoms by impeding TNF-α, IL-1, and IL -6 production [138], as well as reducing NF-B and p38MAPK activation [144, 145], thereby slowing the inflammatory action. As a result, this could diminish the high levels of PICs, which have a negative impact on the outcomes of COVID-19. However, no clinical trials have been conducted that demonstrate losartan's efficacy in COVID-19.

Some medications considered as COVID-19 therapy have previously been employed as antineoplastic agents in leukemias. Among the immunomodulatory antineoplastic medicines, JAK inhibitors and Bruton's tyrosine kinase (BTK) inhibitors have shown potential benefits in COVID-19 patients. Ruxolitinib, a JAK1/2 inhibitor authorised for myeloproliferative neoplasms [146], may be beneficial in COVID-19 hyperinflammation. Preclinical results suggest that ibrutinib (BTK inhibitor) can protect against serious lung injury [147], most likely because of its ability to lower inflammatory mediator levels [148].

Ivermectin is a standard broad-spectrum anti-parasitic agent [149] that has been found to have antiviral activity against various viruses (SARS-CoV-2) *in vitro* and/or *in vivo* [150 - 152], most likely through inhibiting viral protein nuclear trafficking [153]. Furthermore, ivermectin was discovered to have an immunomodulatory profile that altered T- lymphocyte activity and lymphocyte count [154]. Furthermore, this medicine was able to reduce inflammation by lowering the production of various cytokines, including TNF-α, IL- 1, IL-4, IL-5, IL-6, and IL-13 [155, 156]. Hence, this drug can block a range of inflammatory cytokines that play a crucial part in the development of CS, hence lowering COVID-19 consequences.

Clinical trials with hydroxychloroquine (HCQ) and chloroquine (CQ) as COVID-19 preventative treatments are already underway, with inconsistent findings [157]. Preliminary evidence suggests that both drugs are effective against SARS-CoV-2. *In vitro*, both HCQ and CQ drugs have been demonstrated to reduce SARS-Co--2 infection; it is reported that HCQ is more powerful than CQ [158]. Because of its capacity to lower the binding effectiveness of ACE2 in host cells to SARS-CoV-2, HCQ has demonstrated an antiviral profile. Some other studies have looked at the use of HCQ/CQ alone or with other medicines to treat COVID-19, but the results have been weak and inconsistent [157]. As a result, the efficacy of these medications in COVID-19 has not been cleared, so the FDA has revoked their emergency use. Other studies have demonstrated that HCQ, CQ, ivermectin, and nitazoxanide reduce the levels of pro-inflammatory cytokines, hence ameliorating the increased inflammatory process seen in a variety of disorders. These properties of anti-parasitic medications may aid in recovery for patients with COVID- 19. While, the literature suggests that the usage of these medications is inconsistent, more research is needed to assess their efficacy.

GM-CSF medications for COVID-19 patients are under consideration - Otilimab {(anti-GM-CSF) NCT04376684}, Gimsilumab {(anti-GM-CSF) NCT04351243}, Lenzilumab {(anti-GM-CSF) NCT04351152}, TJM2 {(anti-GM-CSF) NCT04341116}, Mavrilimumab {anti-GM-CSFR) NCT04397497}, Namilumab {(anti-GM-CSF)}, Sargramostim{(rhuGM-CSF) NCT04326920)} [106]. Recombinant human GM-CSF (sargramostim) is approved by the FDA for a variety of indications, and it may provide advantages to COVID-19 patients. GM-CSF is required for the maintenance of respiratory function, and also lung sentinel cell-mediated immunity [159]. GM-CSF overexpression in mice hindered hyperoxia-induced lung injury by increasing alveolar wall cell resistance to apoptotic cell death and protecting against secondary bacterial infection [160, 161]. Early raised GM-CSF expression in bronchoalveolar lavage fluid with acute lung injury and ARDS was associated to improved survival, possibly due to improved alveolar macrophage survival [162].

Due to its ability to interact with the pathogenic mechanisms of SARS-CoV-2, colchicines could be helpful in COVID-19 treatment [163]. Colchicines are well used to treat autoinflammatory conditions. Furthermore, colchicine inhibits the formation of ROS and inflammasome activation, resulting in a reduction in inflammatory processes [164, 165]. All of these characteristics may help to alleviate inflammatory symptoms as well as reduce the risk of organ failure. However, whether colchicines are potent drugs against COVID-19 is still doubtful as some studies [166, 167] are not clear about their efficacy in SARS-CoV-2 infection, owing to their weak role in suppressing CS and also cytosolic pH.

TARGETING INDUCTION OF COAGULATION IN COVID-19 PATIENTS

As many as one-third of patients with COVID-19 have thrombotic events. These patients are mainly pulmonary emboli patients and are associated with more serious diseases and higher mortality [168, 169]. However, the research is heterogeneous, and the morbidity depends on the composition of the cohort (for example, the severity of the disease, the characteristics of thrombotic events), the investigations done, and the usage of thromboprophylaxis [170]. For example, venous thromboembolism (VTE) has a high incidence in the viral diseases *viz.* SARS-CoV-1 and H1N1; albeit due to different cohorts and methods, their comparison with COVID-19 patients is not easy [171, 172]. The incidence of VTE in severe COVID-19 is higher than that of the ARDS matched group, which indicates that the high incidence is due to hospitalised patients with mechanisms other than VTE risk factors (for example, reduced mobility and severe illness) [173]. In addition, VTE may not be fully identified in COVID-19 because of the increased incidence during screening investigations.

It is also applicable to other disorders [174]. The smaller lung (micro) thrombosis in patients with COVID-19 may show *in situ* immune thrombosis, which is a mechanism started by the innate immune system and involves interaction with hemostasis [174 - 176]. It is currently uncertain whether COVID-19 -related thrombotic events are because of VTE (conventional), immune thrombosis, or their combination, which is of great significance for diagnosis and management strategies [177]. In Fig. (**3**), the intrinsic pathway of clotting cascade abnormalities in patients with COVID-19 is presented.

COVID-19 Related Coagulopathy

Although the pathophysiology of the hypercoagulable state of COVID-19 is not clear yet, some recommendations have been proposed [178]: disseminated intravascular coagulation (DIC), antiphospholipid syndrome, complement system activation, endothelial dysfunction due to infection, and properties of the virus itself, ascribed towards possible pathophysiology [178 - 181].

Patients with COVID-19 may have mild thrombocytopenia but also prolongation of prothrombination time, increased D-dimer, and elevated fibrinogen. All of these become more noticeable as the severity of the disease increases [177, 182, 183]. Also, COVID-19-associated coagulopathy (CAC) has the same characteristics as sepsis-induced coagulopathy (SIC) and DIC, albeit it is different [184]. Both DIC, as well as SIC, could occur in COVID-19, even though they are common whenever applying diagnostic criteria [184]. Similarly, CAC reports have also been found in SARS-CoV-1 [177].

D-dimer, a fibrin degradation product, is sensitive to fibrinolysis and detects intravascular thrombosis (VTE), but lacks specificity and may be elevated in inflammation and other diseases [185]. An elevated level of D-dimer may occur in COVID-19 and is associated with mortality, independently [186, 187]. Additionally, increased D-dimer may be associated with COVID-19 acute lung injury, which is produced by the decomposition of fibrin in the alveoli deposited in ARDS [187]. Other signatures of coagulation and inflammation in COVID-19 may also be abnormal, including C-reactive protein (CRP), complement system, ferritin, von Willebrand factor (VWF), and cytokines. This implies that there is a complex interaction between the hemostatic system and the immune system that may lead to the prothrombotic phenotypes [177].

Endothelial Dysfunction and COVID-19

The endothelium is a monocellular layer that lines blood arteries, serving as a mechanical barrier between flowing blood and the basement membrane, as well as modulating not only vascular tone but also immunomodulation [188]. Endothelial dysfunction is characterised by increased endothelial activation and decreased endothelium-dependent vasodilation, resulting in a pro-inflammatory, proliferative, and procoagulant state [189]. Patients with disorders (obesity, diabetes, and systemic hypertension, *etc.*) linked with endothelial dysfunction have worse COVID-19 clinical outcomes, and evidence of endothelial dysfunction is also found in the post-mortem of COVID-19 [190, 191]. Endothelial dysfunction may be caused by direct SARS- CoV-2 infection of endothelial cells or by indirect inflammatory consequences [190, 191]. The host serine protease TMPRSS2 aids in the binding of the SARS-CoV-2 spike protein to the ACE2 receptor, which is followed by viral endocytosis and reproduction [192, 193]. Endothelial damage and also viral release induce a strong immunological response, which can lead to more endothelial dysfunction.

Coagulation Test Analysis

Newly diagnosed hospitalised COVID-19 patients or suspected SARS-CoV-2 infection should undergo coagulation tests on admission, including D-dimer, fibrinogen, PT, aPTT, and platelet count tests, which can insight useful prognostic clues [194]. Death-related D-dimer elevations and DIC-related rapid decreases in fibrinogen were observed within 7 to 11 days of symptom onset or 4-10 days after hospitalisation [33, 186]. Time to increase in D-dimer, PT, and aPTT, as well as reductions in fibrinogen and platelet counts, were also consistent with the length of the hospitalizations, which appeared to begin between 7 and 10 days after admission, with D-dimer likely increasing on day 4 [194]. These patients have sepsis and are physiologically critical; changes in coagulation may suggest the development of DIC, which may not be related to the impact of COVID-19 and prolonged hospital stay, mechanical ventilation, re-infection, and ICU causes [194].

Venous Thromboembolic Prophylaxis

Venous thromboembolic (VTE), a polygenic disease that has common and rare genetic variants, includes heritable thrombotic tendency *viz.* factor V Leiden, antithrombin and prothrombin mutations, and protein C/S defects [177]. A genome-wide association study (GWAS) of severe COVID-19 patients revealed the genetic associations in the ABO gene and chromosome 3 locus (3p21.31) across multiple genes (SLC6A20, LZTFL1, CCR9, FYCO1, CXCR6 and XCR1) [177, 195]. Taking into account the high inflammatory state, hospitalised patients with confirmed or suspected COVID-19 should receive drug-based VTE preventive treatment, unless there are specific contraindications [194].

Different settings have increased the preventive anticoagulant dose to an "intermediate intensity" dose of enoxaparin (0.5 mg/kg two times a day), practising a risk fitting strategy, with enhanced doses based on the levels of D-dimer, ICU setting, fibrinogen or other associated factors related to higher risk [194]. The Delphi method consensus document reported that 31.6% of subjects sustained intermediate-intensity doses and 5.2% supported therapeutic doses; another supports optimal VTE use in hospitalised patients with moderate to critically ill COVID-19 and DIC deficiency prophylactic doses [197] and in obese patients, a daily dose of 40 mg enoxaparin is not enough in postoperative situations, because sufficient plasma concentrations are not reached. Higher doses based on body weight, such as 7500 U UFH three times a day or 40mg enoxaparin twice a day, are better tolerated [197, 198]. Increasing the dose of heparin may also be important for preventive treatment to conquer the observed increase in procoagulant proteins- von Willebrand factor, high levels of fibrinogen, and FVIII, which can be seen after orthopaedic joint replacement surgery or not encountered in typical medical patients [199]. Here, individual subject assessments that combine both VTE and bleeding risk factors with clinical evaluation are needed. According to internal audits, Connors JM *et al.* [194] found that compared with patients in the ward, the number of VTEs with 40 mg of enoxaparin per day in the ICU has increased. They said that their institution should increase the preventive dose of anticoagulation therapy for ICU patients [194].

Microvascular Thrombosin

As far as we know, there is no potential antiviral therapeutic for SARS-CoV-2. In cases of severe sepsis, lung injury, or ARDS, proper management should include a review of concomitant infections. Heparin and its derivatives seem to be crucial for VTE management, but previous SIC reports showed limited efficacy. Physiological anticoagulants, such as activated protein C, thrombomodulin, and antithrombin, have previously shown limited efficacy in randomised clinical trials, but they include all patients with sepsis, not just those suffering from toxicosis-related coagulopathy and DIC. However, no significant reduction in antithrombin levels has been found in COVID- 19 infected patients [200].

Although microvascular thrombosis may cause multiorgan failure in patients with long-term infection, early lung injury appears to be caused by inflammation, reactivity, as well as viral effects on lung tissue. Guidelines recommend standard supportive care for sepsis patients. Although the role of anticoagulants or other drugs may lower microvascular thrombosis and potentially end organ dysfunction; no survival benefit has indeed been found in previous trials of sepsis patients, notwithstanding the trend of anticoagulation therapy offering a survival advantage in small subgroups. Patients with sepsis alone, and also patients with sepsis combined with SIC or overt DIC, should continue receiving anticoagulation therapy.

A low-dose of heparin was used in previous sepsis anticoagulation trials [58]. Previous studies on the SARS virus have shown that *in vitro* heparin reduces the infectivity of the SARS-CoV by ~50% [201]. It is not yet clear whether it is due to heparin as a non-specific polyanion that prevents charged spike proteins from binding to their host cell receptors, or due to the specific inhibition of coagulation FXa, which promotes cell entry, on the cleavage of S protein into the activated component [202, 203]. Although it is interesting in theory. However, in the case of SARS, the above processes are not well defined. There is no data on heparin's interaction with SARS-CoV-2, and there is no diagnostic use of heparin to reduce a patient's infectivity.

Clinical Interventions for Therapeutic Anticoagulation

Patients with other anticoagulation indications, such as newly diagnosed VTE, or long-term VTE secondary prevention, mechanical heart valve, and atrial fibrillation, should be prescribed anticoagulant medication at the full dose or one dose similar to the current dose for COVID-19 patients. Due to the short half-life and ability of parenteral administration, LMWH or UFH is superior to direct oral anticoagulants for hospitalised patients, especially critically ill patients. Fibrinogen levels are increased in COVID-19 patients, which is among one of the causes of hypercoagulability and also heparin resistance. As a result, if you have problems with aPTT measurement, you should consider monitoring anti-FXa heparin levels [204].

Due to the difficulties in switching mechanically ventilated patients to CT scanners and the desire to limit staff exposure to COVID-19 patients, the subject of using treatment dose anticoagulation for suspected PE has come up in several ICUs around the world. D-dimer is usually ineffective in these patients due to the large baseline increases. Clinical signs of rapid respiratory relapses, indications of right-heart stress on electrocardiography, or DVT witnessed on lower extremity ultrasonography were used to increase therapeutic-dose anticoagulation. From a clinical point of view, we can't say that therapeutic anticoagulation isn't necessary for that situation.

CONCLUSION

It is clear that medications that directly encounter SARS-CoV-2 would indeed be better treatment options for COVID-19 patients; lowering pro-inflammatory cytokines may also be critical for preventing or lowering the disease's progression and thereby minimising the frequency of serious conditions and hospitalizations. Here, it is important that an upsurge in pro-inflammatory cytokines is linked to a worsening respiratory state as well as hyperinflammation, collectively known as CS. A method that stimulates the innate immune system while decreasing Th1/Th2 inflammation might help in preventing the severe COVID-19 condition and contribute to disease healing. Several medications (summarised in Table **1**) prescribed for the management of COVID-19 have an anti-inflammatory profile, and the majority are responsible for minimising the levels of IL-6 and TNF-α, primal cytokines (key targets for drugs that) handle symptoms of COVID-19. Reducing pro-inflammatory cytokines is also thought to be a major strategy for improving the clinical symptoms in COVID-19 patients and delaying disease progression. The antiviral drugs remdesivir and lopinavir-ritonavir, which are routinely used in the management of HIV- infected individuals, have demonstrated good benefits in COVID-19 patients, lowering symptoms [141]. These medications may have a direct effect on viral replication and thus aid in viral load reduction.

Despite the fact that research into COVID-19-linked VTE and immunothrombosis is expanding, there are still several knowledge gaps. Dissecting as well as describing the particular effects of SARS-CoV-2 on thrombosis is a continuing topic of research that is critical for guiding therapies. According to Loo J *et al.* [81], future COVID-19 research should focus on a) small pulmonary thrombosis, whether representing VTE, immunothrombosis, or a combination of the two; (b) whether diagnostic practices, such as radiological and biochemical, can correctly diagnose and clearly distinguish between VTE and immunothrombosis; (c) how the risk of immunothrombosis can be measured and predicted; and (d) the role of anticoagulation in immunothrombosis. The majority of COVID-19 studies are cross-sectional and/or observational with severely ill patients (with lower samples). Randomized control trials with a large sample size are needed to gain a better understanding of immunothrombosis and pro-inflammatory cytokines targeting repurposed drugs.

CONSENT FOR PUBLICATION

Not applicable.

CONFLICT OF INTEREST

The author declares no conflict of interest, financial or otherwise.

ACKNOWLEDGEMENTS

Declared none.

REFERENCES

[1] Alam M. RM P. Ivermectin as pre-exposure prophylaxis for COVID 19 among healthcare providers in a selected tertiary hospital in Dhaka an observational study. Eur J Med Health Sci 2020; 2: 1-5.

[2] https://www.worldometers.info/coronavirus/

[3] Naqvi AAT, Fatima K, Mohammad T, *et al.* Insights into SARS-CoV-2 genome, structure, evolution, pathogenesis and therapies: Structural genomics approach. Biochim Biophys Acta Mol Basis Dis 2020; 1866(10): 165878.
[http://dx.doi.org/10.1016/j.bbadis.2020.165878] [PMID: 32544429]

[4] Cui J, Li F, Shi ZL. Origin and evolution of pathogenic coronaviruses. Nat Rev Microbiol 2019; 17(3): 181-92.

[http://dx.doi.org/10.1038/s41579-018-0118-9] [PMID: 30531947]

[5]   Guo YR, Cao QD, Hong ZS, *et al.* The origin, transmission and clinical therapies on coronavirus disease 2019 (COVID-19) outbreak – an update on the status. Mil Med Res 2020; 7(1): 11.
[http://dx.doi.org/10.1186/s40779-020-00240-0] [PMID: 32169119]

[6]   Wiersinga WJ, Rhodes A, Cheng AC, Peacock SJ, Prescott HC. Pathophysiology, Transmission, Diagnosis, and Treatment of Coronavirus Disease 2019 (COVID-19). JAMA 2020; 324(8): 782-93.
[http://dx.doi.org/10.1001/jama.2020.12839] [PMID: 32648899]

[7]   Zhong NS, Zheng BJ, Li YM, *et al.* Epidemiology and cause of severe acute respiratory syndrome (SARS) in Guangdong, People's Republic of China, in February, 2003. Lancet 2003; 362(9393): 1353-8.
[http://dx.doi.org/10.1016/S0140-6736(03)14630-2] [PMID: 14585636]

[8]   Guarner J. Three emerging coronaviruses in two decades: the story of SARS, MERS, and now COVID-19. Am J Clin Pathol 2020; 153(4): 420-1.
[http://dx.doi.org/10.1093/ajcp/aqaa029] [PMID: 32053148]

[9]   Zhou P, Yang XL, Wang XG, *et al.* A pneumonia outbreak associated with a new coronavirus of probable bat origin. Nature 2020; 579(7798): 270-3.
[http://dx.doi.org/10.1038/s41586-020-2012-7] [PMID: 32015507]

[10]   Hu B, Guo H, Zhou P, Shi ZL. Characteristics of SARS-CoV-2 and COVID-19. Nat Rev Microbiol 2021; 19(3): 141-54.
[http://dx.doi.org/10.1038/s41579-020-00459-7] [PMID: 33024307]

[11]   Lan J, Ge J, Yu J, *et al.* Structure of the SARS-CoV-2 spike receptor-binding domain bound to the ACE2 receptor. Nature 2020; 581(7807): 215-20.
[http://dx.doi.org/10.1038/s41586-020-2180-5] [PMID: 32225176]

[12]   Meyerowitz EA, Richterman A, Gandhi RT, Sax PE. Transmission of SARS-CoV-2: a review of viral, host, and environmental factors. Ann Intern Med 2021; 174(1): 69-79.
[http://dx.doi.org/10.7326/M20-5008] [PMID: 32941052]

[13]   da Costa VG, Moreli ML, Saivish MV. The emergence of SARS, MERS and novel SARS-2 coronaviruses in the 21st century. Arch Virol 2020; 165(7): 1517-26.
[http://dx.doi.org/10.1007/s00705-020-04628-0] [PMID: 32322993]

[14]   Shang J, Ye G, Shi K, *et al.* Structural basis of receptor recognition by SARS-CoV-2. Nature 2020; 581(7807): 221-4.
[http://dx.doi.org/10.1038/s41586-020-2179-y] [PMID: 32225175]

[15]   Zhang L, Lin D, Sun X, *et al.* Crystal structure of SARS-CoV-2 main protease provides a basis for design of improved α-ketoamide inhibitors. Science 2020; 368(6489): 409-12.
[http://dx.doi.org/10.1126/science.abb3405] [PMID: 32198291]

[16]   Walls AC, Park YJ, Tortorici MA, Wall A, McGuire AT, Veesler D. Structure, function, and antigenicity of the SARS-CoV-2 spike glycoprotein. Cell 2020; 181(2): 281-292.e6.
[http://dx.doi.org/10.1016/j.cell.2020.02.058] [PMID: 32155444]

[17]   Siu YL, Teoh KT, Lo J, *et al.* The M, E, and N structural proteins of the severe acute respiratory syndrome coronavirus are required for efficient assembly, trafficking, and release of virus-like particles. J Virol 2008; 82(22): 11318-30.
[http://dx.doi.org/10.1128/JVI.01052-08] [PMID: 18753196]

[18]   Satarker S, Nampoothiri M. Structural proteins in severe acute respiratory syndrome coronavirus-2. Arch Med Res 2020; 51(6): 482-91.
[http://dx.doi.org/10.1016/j.arcmed.2020.05.012] [PMID: 32493627]

[19]   Huang Y, Yang C, Xu X, Xu W, Liu S. Structural and functional properties of SARS-CoV-2 spike protein: potential antivirus drug development for COVID-19. Acta Pharmacol Sin 2020; 41(9): 1141-9.

[http://dx.doi.org/10.1038/s41401-020-0485-4] [PMID: 32747721]

[20]   Duan L, Zheng Q, Zhang H, Niu Y, Lou Y, Wang H. The SARS-CoV-2 spike glycoprotein biosynthesis, structure, function, and antigenicity: Implications for the design of spike-based vaccine immunogens. Front Immunol 2020; 11: 576622.
[http://dx.doi.org/10.3389/fimmu.2020.576622] [PMID: 33117378]

[21]   Hu Y, Wen J, Tang L, *et al.* The M protein of SARS-CoV: basic structural and immunological properties. Genomics Proteomics Bioinformatics 2003; 1(2): 118-30.
[http://dx.doi.org/10.1016/S1672-0229(03)01016-7] [PMID: 15626342]

[22]   Singh Tomar PP, Arkin IT. SARS-CoV-2 E protein is a potential ion channel that can be inhibited by Gliclazide and Memantine. Biochem Biophys Res Commun 2020; 530(1): 10-4.
[http://dx.doi.org/10.1016/j.bbrc.2020.05.206] [PMID: 32828269]

[23]   Sarkar M, Saha S. Structural insight into the role of novel SARS-CoV-2 E protein: A potential target for vaccine development and other therapeutic strategies. PLoS One 2020; 15(8): e0237300.
[http://dx.doi.org/10.1371/journal.pone.0237300] [PMID: 32785274]

[24]   Dutta NK, Mazumdar K, Gordy JT. The nucleocapsid protein of SARS–CoV-2: a target for vaccine development. J Virol 2020; 94(13): e00647-20.
[http://dx.doi.org/10.1128/JVI.00647-20] [PMID: 32546606]

[25]   Klausegger A, Strobl B, Regl G, Kaser A, Luytjes W, Vlasak R. Identification of a coronavirus hemagglutinin-esterase with a substrate specificity different from those of influenza C virus and bovine coronavirus. J Virol 1999; 73(5): 3737-43.
[http://dx.doi.org/10.1128/JVI.73.5.3737-3743.1999] [PMID: 10196267]

[26]   Lopez-Rincon A, Perez-Romero CA, Tonda A, *et al.* Design of specific primer sets for the detection of B. 1.1. 7, B.1.351 and 1.BioRxiv 2021;

[27]   Vrancken B, Dellicour S, Smith DM, Chaillon A. Phylogenetic analyses of SARS-CoV-2 B. 1.1. 7 lineage suggest a single origin followed by multiple exportation events *versus* convergent evolution. bioRxiv 2021.

[28]   Emerging SARS-CoV-2 variants 2021.https://www.cdc.gov/coronavirus/2019-ncov/more/science-a-d-research/scientific-brief-emerging-variants.html

[29]   Starr TN, Greaney AJ, Addetia A, *et al.* Prospective mapping of viral mutations that escape antibodies used to treat COVID-19. Science 2021; 371(6531): 850-4.
[http://dx.doi.org/10.1126/science.abf9302] [PMID: 33495308]

[30]   Simmons G, Zmora P, Gierer S, Heurich A, Pöhlmann S. Proteolytic activation of the SARS-coronavirus spike protein: Cutting enzymes at the cutting edge of antiviral research. Antiviral Res 2013; 100(3): 605-14.
[http://dx.doi.org/10.1016/j.antiviral.2013.09.028] [PMID: 24121034]

[31]   Heurich A, Hofmann-Winkler H, Gierer S, Liepold T, Jahn O, Pöhlmann S. TMPRSS2 and ADAM17 cleave ACE2 differentially and only proteolysis by TMPRSS2 augments entry driven by the severe acute respiratory syndrome coronavirus spike protein. J Virol 2014; 88(2): 1293-307.
[http://dx.doi.org/10.1128/JVI.02202-13] [PMID: 24227843]

[32]   Fehr AR, Perlman S. Coronaviruses: an overview of their replication and pathogenesis. Methods Mol Biol 2015; 1282: 1-23.
[http://dx.doi.org/10.1007/978-1-4939-2438-7_1] [PMID: 25720466]

[33]   Zhou F, Yu T, Du R, *et al.* Clinical course and risk factors for mortality of adult inpatients with COVID-19 in Wuhan, China: a retrospective cohort study. Lancet 2020; 395(10229): 1054-62.
[http://dx.doi.org/10.1016/S0140-6736(20)30566-3] [PMID: 32171076]

[34]   Chen Y, Shan K, Qian W. Asians and Other Races Express Similar Levels of and Share the Same Genetic Polymorphisms of the SARS-CoV-2 Cell-Entry Receptor. Preprints 2020; 2020020258.
[http://dx.doi.org/10.20944/preprints202002.0258.v1]

[35]   Zhang JM, An J. Cytokines, inflammation, and pain. Int Anesthesiol Clin 2007; 45(2): 27-37.
[http://dx.doi.org/10.1097/AIA.0b013e318034194e] [PMID: 17426506]

[36]   Clark IA, Virelizier JL, Carswell EA, Wood PR. Possible importance of macrophage-derived mediators in acute malaria. Infect Immun 1981; 32(3): 1058-66.
[http://dx.doi.org/10.1128/iai.32.3.1058-1066.1981] [PMID: 6166564]

[37]   Clark IA. Suggested importance of monokines in pathophysiology of endotoxin shock and malaria. Klin Wochenschr 1982; 60(14): 756-8.
[http://dx.doi.org/10.1007/BF01716573] [PMID: 6181289]

[38]   Makhija R, Kingsnorth AN. Cytokine storm in acute pancreatitis. J Hepatobiliary Pancreat Surg 2002; 9(4): 401-10.
[http://dx.doi.org/10.1007/s005340200049] [PMID: 12483260]

[39]   Jahrling PB, Hensley LE, Martinez MJ, *et al.* Exploring the potential of variola virus infection of cynomolgus macaques as a model for human smallpox. Proc Natl Acad Sci USA 2004; 101(42): 15196-200.
[http://dx.doi.org/10.1073/pnas.0405954101] [PMID: 15477589]

[40]   Yuen KY, Wong SS. Human infection by avian influenza A H5N1. Hong Kong Med J 2005; 11(3): 189-99.
[PMID: 15951584]

[41]   Fara A, Mitrev Z, Rosalia RA, Assas BM. Cytokine storm and COVID-19: a chronicle of pro-inflammatory cytokines. Open Biol 2020; 10(9): 200160.
[http://dx.doi.org/10.1098/rsob.200160] [PMID: 32961074]

[42]   Zhao L, Cao YJ. Engineered T cell therapy for cancer in the clinic. Front Immunol 2019; 10: 2250.
[http://dx.doi.org/10.3389/fimmu.2019.02250] [PMID: 31681259]

[43]   Suntharalingam G, Perry MR, Ward S, *et al.* Cytokine storm in a phase 1 trial of the anti-CD28 monoclonal antibody TGN1412. N Engl J Med 2006; 355(10): 1018-28.
[http://dx.doi.org/10.1056/NEJMoa063842] [PMID: 16908486]

[44]   Hansel TT, Kropshofer H, Singer T, Mitchell JA, George AJT. The safety and side effects of monoclonal antibodies. Nat Rev Drug Discov 2010; 9(4): 325-38.
[http://dx.doi.org/10.1038/nrd3003] [PMID: 20305665]

[45]   Honjo O, Kubo T, Sugaya F, *et al.* Severe cytokine release syndrome resulting in purpura fulminans despite successful response to nivolumab therapy in a patient with pleomorphic carcinoma of the lung: a case report. J Immunother Cancer 2019; 7(1): 97.
[http://dx.doi.org/10.1186/s40425-019-0582-4] [PMID: 30944043]

[46]   Ceschi A, Noseda R, Palin K, Verhamme K. Immune checkpoint inhibitor-related cytokine release syndrome: analysis of WHO global pharmacovigilance database. Front Pharmacol 2020; 11: 557.
[http://dx.doi.org/10.3389/fphar.2020.00557] [PMID: 32425791]

[47]   Bakacs T, Mehrishi JN, Moss RW. Ipilimumab (Yervoy) and the TGN1412 catastrophe. Immunobiology 2012; 217(6): 583-9.
[http://dx.doi.org/10.1016/j.imbio.2011.07.005] [PMID: 21821307]

[48]   Huang KJ, Su IJ, Theron M, *et al.* An interferon-?-related cytokine storm in SARS patients. J Med Virol 2005; 75(2): 185-94.
[http://dx.doi.org/10.1002/jmv.20255] [PMID: 15602737]

[49]   Sinha P, Matthay MA, Calfee CS. Is a"cytokine storm" relevant to COVID-19? JAMA Intern Med 2020; 180(9): 1152-4.
[http://dx.doi.org/10.1001/jamainternmed.2020.3313] [PMID: 32602883]

[50]   Moore JB, June CH. Cytokine release syndrome in severe COVID-19. Science 2020; 368(6490): 473-4.

[http://dx.doi.org/10.1126/science.abb8925] [PMID: 32303591]

[51]   Horby P, Lim WS, Emberson JR, *et al.* Dexamethasone in Hospitalized Patients with Covid-19. N Engl J Med 2021; 384(8): 693-704.
[http://dx.doi.org/10.1056/NEJMoa2021436] [PMID: 32678530]

[52]   Huang C, Wang Y, Li X, *et al.* Clinical features of patients infected with 2019 novel coronavirus in Wuhan, China. Lancet 2020; 395(10223): 497-506.
[http://dx.doi.org/10.1016/S0140-6736(20)30183-5] [PMID: 31986264]

[53]   Zhu Z, Cai T, Fan L, *et al.* Clinical value of immune-inflammatory parameters to assess the severity of coronavirus disease 2019. Int J Infect Dis 2020; 95: 332-9.
[http://dx.doi.org/10.1016/j.ijid.2020.04.041] [PMID: 32334118]

[54]   Del Valle DM, Kim-Schulze S, Huang HH, *et al.* An inflammatory cytokine signature predicts COVID-19 severity and survival. Nat Med 2020; 26(10): 1636-43.
[http://dx.doi.org/10.1038/s41591-020-1051-9] [PMID: 32839624]

[55]   Mathew D, Giles JR, Baxter AE, *et al.* Deep immune profiling of COVID-19 patients reveals distinct immunotypes with therapeutic implications. Science 2020; 369(6508): eabc8511.
[http://dx.doi.org/10.1126/science.abc8511] [PMID: 32669297]

[56]   Caricchio R, Gallucci M, Dass C, *et al.* Preliminary predictive criteria for COVID-19 cytokine storm. Ann Rheum Dis 2021; 80(1): 88-95.
[http://dx.doi.org/10.1136/annrheumdis-2020-218323] [PMID: 32978237]

[57]   Bindoli S, Felicetti M, Sfriso P, Doria A. The amount of cytokine-release defines different shades of Sars-Cov2 infection. Exp Biol Med (Maywood) 2020; 245(11): 970-6.
[http://dx.doi.org/10.1177/1535370220928964] [PMID: 32460624]

[58]   Sarzi-Puttini P, Giorgi V, Sirotti S, *et al.* COVID-19, cytokines and immunosuppression: what can we learn from severe acute respiratory syndrome? Clin Exp Rheumatol 2020; 38(2): 337-42.
[http://dx.doi.org/10.55563/clinexprheumatol/xcdary] [PMID: 32202240]

[59]   Murakami M, Kamimura D, Hirano T. Pleiotropy and specificity: insights from the interleukin 6 family of cytokines. Immunity 2019; 50(4): 812-31.
[http://dx.doi.org/10.1016/j.immuni.2019.03.027] [PMID: 30995501]

[60]   Cooke A, Ferraccioli GF, Herrmann M, *et al.* Induction and protection of autoimmune rheumatic diseases. The role of infections. Clin Exp Rheumatol 2008; 26(1) (Suppl. 48): S1-7.
[PMID: 18570747]

[61]   Takeda K, Akira S. TLR signaling pathways. In Seminars in Immunology. Academic Press 2004; 16: pp. (1)3-9.
[http://dx.doi.org/10.1016/j.smim.2003.10.003]

[62]   Garcia Borrega J, Gödel P, Rüger MA, *et al.* In the eye of the storm: immune-mediated toxicities associated with CAR-T cell therapy. HemaSphere 2019; 3(2): e191.
[http://dx.doi.org/10.1097/HS9.0000000000000191] [PMID: 31723828]

[63]   Li X, Geng M, Peng Y, Meng L, Lu S. Molecular immune pathogenesis and diagnosis of COVID-19. J Pharm Anal 2020; 10(2): 102-8.
[http://dx.doi.org/10.1016/j.jpha.2020.03.001] [PMID: 32282863]

[64]   Zhang C, Wu Z, Li JW, Zhao H, Wang GQ. Cytokine release syndrome in severe COVID-19: interleukin-6 receptor antagonist tocilizumab may be the key to reduce mortality. Int J Antimicrob Agents 2020; 55(5): 105954.
[http://dx.doi.org/10.1016/j.ijantimicag.2020.105954] [PMID: 32234467]

[65]   Leiva-Juárez MM, Kolls JK, Evans SE. Lung epithelial cells: therapeutically inducible effectors of antimicrobial defense. Mucosal Immunol 2018; 11(1): 21-34.
[http://dx.doi.org/10.1038/mi.2017.71] [PMID: 28812547]

[66]   McGonagle D, Sharif K, O'Regan A, Bridgewood C. The role of cytokines including interleukin-6 in COVID-19 induced pneumonia and macrophage activation syndrome-like disease. Autoimmun Rev 2020; 19(6): 102537.
[http://dx.doi.org/10.1016/j.autrev.2020.102537] [PMID: 32251717]

[67]   Wan S, Yi Q, Fan S, *et al.* Characteristics of lymphocyte subsets and cytokines in peripheral blood of 123 hospitalized patients with 2019 novel coronavirus pneumonia (NCP) MedRxiv 2020; 10.20021832.
[http://dx.doi.org/10.1101/2020.02.10.20021832]

[68]   Wypasek E, Undas A, Sniezek-Maciejewska M, *et al.* The increased plasma C-reactive protein and interleukin-6 levels in patients undergoing coronary artery bypass grafting surgery are associated with the interleukin-6–174G > C gene polymorphism. Ann Clin Biochem 2010; 47(4): 343-9.
[http://dx.doi.org/10.1258/acb.2010.090305] [PMID: 20592333]

[69]   Rosalia RA, Arenas-Ramirez N, Bouchaud G, Raeber ME, Boyman O. Use of enhanced interleukin-2 formulations for improved immunotherapy against cancer. Curr Opin Chem Biol 2014; 23: 39-46.
[http://dx.doi.org/10.1016/j.cbpa.2014.09.006] [PMID: 25271022]

[70]   Herrmann F, Oster W, Meuer SC, Lindemann A, Mertelsmann RH. Interleukin 1 stimulates T lymphocytes to produce granulocyte-monocyte colony-stimulating factor. J Clin Invest 1988; 81(5): 1415-8.
[http://dx.doi.org/10.1172/JCI113471] [PMID: 2452833]

[71]   Lichtman AH, Chin J, Schmidt JA, Abbas AK. Role of interleukin 1 in the activation of T lymphocytes. Proc Natl Acad Sci USA 1988; 85(24): 9699-703.
[http://dx.doi.org/10.1073/pnas.85.24.9699] [PMID: 3264404]

[72]   Taylor-Robinson AW, Phillips RS. Expression of the IL-1 receptor discriminates Th2 from Th1 cloned CD4+ T cells specific for Plasmodium chabaudi. Immunology 1994; 81(2): 216-21.
[PMID: 7512528]

[73]   Nakae S, Komiyama Y, Yokoyama H, *et al.* IL-1 is required for allergen-specific Th2 cell activation and the development of airway hypersensitivity response. Int Immunol 2003; 15(4): 483-90.
[http://dx.doi.org/10.1093/intimm/dxg054] [PMID: 12663678]

[74]   Pedersen SF, Ho YC. SARS-CoV-2: a storm is raging. J Clin Invest 2020; 130(5): 2202-5.
[http://dx.doi.org/10.1172/JCI137647] [PMID: 32217834]

[75]   Dienz O, Rincon M. The effects of IL-6 on CD4 T cell responses. Clin Immunol 2009; 130(1): 27-33.
[http://dx.doi.org/10.1016/j.clim.2008.08.018] [PMID: 18845487]

[76]   Ivanov II, McKenzie BS, Zhou L, *et al.* The orphan nuclear receptor RORgammat directs the differentiation program of proinflammatory IL-17+ T helper cells. Cell 2006; 126(6): 1121-33.
[http://dx.doi.org/10.1016/j.cell.2006.07.035] [PMID: 16990136]

[77]   Yang R, Masters AR, Fortner KA, *et al.* IL-6 promotes the differentiation of a subset of naive CD8+ T cells into IL-21–producing B helper CD8+ T cells. J Exp Med 2016; 213(11): 2281-91.
[http://dx.doi.org/10.1084/jem.20160417] [PMID: 27670591]

[78]   Dominitzki S, Fantini MC, Neufert C, *et al.* Cutting edge: trans-signaling *via* the soluble IL-6R abrogates the induction of FoxP3 in naive CD4+CD25 T cells. J Immunol 2007; 179(4): 2041-5.
[http://dx.doi.org/10.4049/jimmunol.179.4.2041] [PMID: 17675459]

[79]   Garlanda C, Dinarello CA, Mantovani A. The interleukin-1 family: back to the future. Immunity 2013; 39(6): 1003-18.
[http://dx.doi.org/10.1016/j.immuni.2013.11.010] [PMID: 24332029]

[80]   Martinon F, Pétrilli V, Mayor A, Tardivel A, Tschopp J. Gout-associated uric acid crystals activate the NALP3 inflammasome. Nature 2006; 440(7081): 237-41.
[http://dx.doi.org/10.1038/nature04516] [PMID: 16407889]

[81] Frank D, Vince JE. Pyroptosis *versus* necroptosis: similarities, differences, and crosstalk. Cell Death Differ 2019; 26(1): 99-114.
[http://dx.doi.org/10.1038/s41418-018-0212-6] [PMID: 30341423]

[82] Netea MG, Kullberg BJ, Verschueren I, Meer JWMV. Interleukin-18 induces production of proinflammatory cytokines in mice: no intermediate role for the cytokines of the tumor necrosis factor family and interleukin-1β. Eur J Immunol 2000; 30(10): 3057-60.
[http://dx.doi.org/10.1002/1521-4141(200010)30:10<3057::AID-IMMU3057>3.0.CO;2-P] [PMID: 11069090]

[83] Dinarello CA, Novick D, Kim S, Kaplanski G. Interleukin-18 and IL-18 binding protein. Front Immunol 2013; 4: 289.
[http://dx.doi.org/10.3389/fimmu.2013.00289] [PMID: 24115947]

[84] Mazodier K, Marin V, Novick D, *et al.* Severe imbalance of IL-18/IL-18BP in patients with secondary hemophagocytic syndrome. Blood 2005; 106(10): 3483-9.
[http://dx.doi.org/10.1182/blood-2005-05-1980] [PMID: 16020503]

[85] Novick D, Kim S, Kaplanski G, Dinarello CA. Interleukin-18, more than a Th1 cytokine. In Seminars in Immunology. Academic Press 2013; 25: pp. (6)439-48.
[http://dx.doi.org/10.1016/j.smim.2013.10.014]

[86] Ruan Q, Yang K, Wang W, Jiang L, Song J. Correction to: Clinical predictors of mortality due to COVID-19 based on an analysis of data of 150 patients from Wuhan, China. Intensive Care Med 2020; 46(6): 1294-7.
[http://dx.doi.org/10.1007/s00134-020-06028-z] [PMID: 32253449]

[87] Lin L, Lu L, Cao W, Li T. Hypothesis for potential pathogenesis of SARS-CoV-2 infection–a review of immune changes in patients with viral pneumonia. Emerg Microbes Infect 2020; 9(1): 727-32.
[http://dx.doi.org/10.1080/22221751.2020.1746199] [PMID: 32196410]

[88] Herold T, Jurinovic V, Arnreich C, *et al.* Elevated levels of IL-6 and CRP predict the need for mechanical ventilation in COVID-19. J Allergy Clin Immunol 2020; 146(1): 128-136.e4.
[http://dx.doi.org/10.1016/j.jaci.2020.05.008] [PMID: 32425269]

[89] Zheng HY, Zhang M, Yang CX, *et al.* Elevated exhaustion levels and reduced functional diversity of T cells in peripheral blood may predict severe progression in COVID-19 patients. Cell Mol Immunol 2020; 17(5): 541-3.
[http://dx.doi.org/10.1038/s41423-020-0401-3] [PMID: 32203186]

[90] Prompetchara E, Ketloy C, Palaga T. Immune responses in COVID-19 and potential vaccines: Lessons learned from SARS and MERS epidemic. Asian Pac J Allergy Immunol 2020; 38(1): 1-9.
[PMID: 32105090]

[91] Chen G, Wu D, Guo W, *et al.* Clinical and immunological features of severe and moderate coronavirus disease 2019. J Clin Invest 2020; 130(5): 2620-9.
[http://dx.doi.org/10.1172/JCI137244] [PMID: 32217835]

[92] Fajgenbaum DC, June CH. Cytokine Storm. N Engl J Med 2020; 383(23): 2255-73.
[http://dx.doi.org/10.1056/NEJMra2026131] [PMID: 33264547]

[93] Shi Y, Wang Y, Shao C, *et al.* COVID-19 infection: the perspectives on immune responses. Cell Death Differ 2020; 27(5): 1451-4.
[http://dx.doi.org/10.1038/s41418-020-0530-3] [PMID: 32205856]

[94] Lee SMY, Cheung CY, Nicholls JM, *et al.* Hyperinduction of cyclooxygenase-2-mediated proinflammatory cascade: a mechanism for the pathogenesis of avian influenza H5N1 infection. J Infect Dis 2008; 198(4): 525-35.
[http://dx.doi.org/10.1086/590499] [PMID: 18613795]

[95] Rosalia RA, Štěpánek I, Polláková V, *et al.* Administration of anti-CD25 mAb leads to impaired α-galactosylceramide-mediated induction of IFN-γ production in a murine model. Immunobiology 2013;

218(6): 851-9.
[http://dx.doi.org/10.1016/j.imbio.2012.10.012] [PMID: 23182710]

[96]　Parkin J, Cohen B. An overview of the immune system. Lancet 2001; 357(9270): 1777-89.
　　　 [http://dx.doi.org/10.1016/S0140-6736(00)04904-7] [PMID: 11403834]

[97]　Zheng M, Gao Y, Wang G, *et al.* Functional exhaustion of antiviral lymphocytes in COVID-19 patients. Cell Mol Immunol 2020; 17(5): 533-5.
　　　 [http://dx.doi.org/10.1038/s41423-020-0402-2] [PMID: 32203188]

[98]　Mahallawi WH, Khabour OF, Zhang Q, Makhdoum HM, Suliman BA. MERS-CoV infection in humans is associated with a pro-inflammatory Th1 and Th17 cytokine profile. Cytokine 2018; 104: 8-13.
　　　 [http://dx.doi.org/10.1016/j.cyto.2018.01.025] [PMID: 29414327]

[99]　Wong CK, Lam CWK, Wu AKL, *et al.* Plasma inflammatory cytokines and chemokines in severe acute respiratory syndrome. Clin Exp Immunol 2004; 136(1): 95-103.
　　　 [http://dx.doi.org/10.1111/j.1365-2249.2004.02415.x] [PMID: 15030519]

[100]　Bonaventura A, Vecchié A, Wang TS, *et al.* Targeting GM-CSF in COVID-19 pneumonia: rationale and strategies. Front Immunol 2020; 11: 1625.
　　　 [http://dx.doi.org/10.3389/fimmu.2020.01625] [PMID: 32719685]

[101]　Shakoory B, Carcillo JA, Chatham WW, *et al.* Interleukin-1 receptor blockade is associated with reduced mortality in sepsis patients with features of the macrophage activation syndrome: Re-analysis of a prior Phase III trial. Crit Care Med 2016; 44(2): 275-81.
　　　 [http://dx.doi.org/10.1097/CCM.0000000000001402] [PMID: 26584195]

[102]　Toldo S, Abbate A. The NLRP3 inflammasome in acute myocardial infarction. Nat Rev Cardiol 2018; 15(4): 203-14.
　　　 [http://dx.doi.org/10.1038/nrcardio.2017.161] [PMID: 29143812]

[103]　Dixon DL, Van Tassell BW, Vecchié A, *et al.* Cardiovascular considerations in treating patients with coronavirus disease 2019 (COVID-19). J Cardiovasc Pharmacol 2020; 75(5): 359-67.
　　　 [http://dx.doi.org/10.1097/FJC.0000000000000836] [PMID: 32282502]

[104]　Dinarello CA. The IL-1 family of cytokines and receptors in rheumatic diseases. Nat Rev Rheumatol 2019; 15(10): 612-32.
　　　 [http://dx.doi.org/10.1038/s41584-019-0277-8] [PMID: 31515542]

[105]　Lang FM, Lee KMC, Teijaro JR, Becher B, Hamilton JA. GM-CSF-based treatments in COVID-19: reconciling opposing therapeutic approaches. Nat Rev Immunol 2020; 20(8): 507-14.
　　　 [http://dx.doi.org/10.1038/s41577-020-0357-7] [PMID: 32576980]

[106]　Ashburn TT, Thor KB. Drug repositioning: identifying and developing new uses for existing drugs. Nat Rev Drug Discov 2004; 3(8): 673-83.
　　　 [http://dx.doi.org/10.1038/nrd1468] [PMID: 15286734]

[107]　Pushpakom S, Iorio F, Eyers PA, *et al.* Drug repurposing: progress, challenges and recommendations. Nat Rev Drug Discov 2019; 18(1): 41-58.
　　　 [http://dx.doi.org/10.1038/nrd.2018.168] [PMID: 30310233]

[108]　Monteiro WM, Brito-Sousa JD, Baía-da-Silva D, *et al.* Driving forces for COVID-19 clinical trials using chloroquine: the need to choose the right research questions and outcomes. Rev Soc Bras Med Trop 2020; 53: e20200155.
　　　 [http://dx.doi.org/10.1590/0037-8682-0155-2020] [PMID: 32267301]

[109]　Heimfarth L, Serafini MR, Martins-Filho PR, Quintans JSS, Quintans-Júnior LJ. Drug repurposing and cytokine management in response to COVID-19: A review. Int Immunopharmacol 2020; 88: 106947.
　　　 [http://dx.doi.org/10.1016/j.intimp.2020.106947] [PMID: 32919216]

[110]　Gonçalves A, Bertrand J, Ke R. Timing of antiviral treatment initiation is critical to reduce SARS-

Cov-2 viral load. medRxiv 2020; 2020.04.
[http://dx.doi.org/10.1101/2020.04.04.20047886]

[111] Wang Y, Zhang D, Du G, *et al.* Remdesivir in adults with severe COVID-19: a randomised, double-blind, placebo-controlled, multicentre trial. Lancet 2020; 395(10236): 1569-78.
[http://dx.doi.org/10.1016/S0140-6736(20)31022-9] [PMID: 32423584]

[112] Chaves OA, Sacramento CQ, Ferreira AC, *et al.* Atazanavir is a competitive inhibitor of SARS-CoV-2 Mpro, impairing variants replication *in vitro* and *in vivo*. Pharmaceuticals (Basel) 2021; 15(1): 21.
[http://dx.doi.org/10.3390/ph15010021] [PMID: 35056078]

[113] Tanaka T, Kamiyama T, Daikoku T, *et al.* T-705 (Favipiravir) suppresses tumor necrosis factor α production in response to influenza virus infection: A beneficial feature of T-705 as an anti-influenza drug. Acta Virol 2017; 61(1): 48-55.
[http://dx.doi.org/10.4149/av_2017_01_48] [PMID: 28105854]

[114] Fagone P, Mangano K, Quattrocchi C, *et al.* Effects of NO-Hybridization on the Immunomodulatory Properties of the HIV Protease Inhibitors Lopinavir and Ritonavir. Basic Clin Pharmacol Toxicol 2015; 117(5): 306-15.
[http://dx.doi.org/10.1111/bcpt.12414] [PMID: 25903922]

[115] Wang Y, Ding Y, Yang C, *et al.* Inhibition of the infectivity and inflammatory response of influenza virus by Arbidol hydrochloride *in vitro* and *in vivo* (mice and ferret). Biomed Pharmacother 2017; 91: 393-401.
[http://dx.doi.org/10.1016/j.biopha.2017.04.091] [PMID: 28475918]

[116] Mahevas M, Tran V-T, Roumier M, Chabrol A, Paule R, Guillaud C. No evidence of clinical efficacy of hydroxychloroquine in patients hospitalized for COVID-19 infection with oxygen requirement: results of a study using routinely collected data to emulate a target trial MedRxiv 2020; 20060699.

[117] Zhang B, Zhou X, Zhu C, *et al.* Immune phenotyping based on the neutrophil-to-lymphocyte ratio and IgG level predicts disease severity and outcome for patients with COVID-19. Front Mol Biosci 2020; 7: 157.
[http://dx.doi.org/10.3389/fmolb.2020.00157] [PMID: 32719810]

[118] Qin C, Zhou L, Hu Z, *et al.* Dysregulation of Immune Response in Patients With Coronavirus 2019 (COVID-19) in Wuhan, China. Clin Infect Dis 2020; 71(15): 762-8.
[http://dx.doi.org/10.1093/cid/ciaa248] [PMID: 32161940]

[119] Duret PM, Sebbag E, Mallick A, Gravier S, Spielmann L, Messer L. Recovery from COVID-19 in a patient with spondyloarthritis treated with TNF-alpha inhibitor etanercept. Ann Rheum Dis 2020; 79(9): 1251-2.
[http://dx.doi.org/10.1136/annrheumdis-2020-217362] [PMID: 32354772]

[120] Bennardo F, Buffone C, Giudice A. New therapeutic opportunities for COVID-19 patients with Tocilizumab: Possible correlation of interleukin-6 receptor inhibitors with osteonecrosis of the jaws. Oral Oncol 2020; 106: 104659.
[http://dx.doi.org/10.1016/j.oraloncology.2020.104659] [PMID: 32209313]

[121] Giacomelli R, Sota J, Ruscitti P, *et al.* The treatment of adult-onset Still's disease with anakinra, a recombinant human IL-1 receptor antagonist: a systematic review of literature. Clin Exp Rheumatol 2021; 39(1): 187-95.
[http://dx.doi.org/10.55563/clinexprheumatol/fsq5vq] [PMID: 32452353]

[122] Migita K, Izumi Y, Torigoshi T, *et al.* Inhibition of Janus kinase/signal transducer and activator of transcription (JAK/STAT) signalling pathway in rheumatoid synovial fibroblasts using small molecule compounds. Clin Exp Immunol 2013; 174(3): 356-63.
[http://dx.doi.org/10.1111/cei.12190] [PMID: 23968543]

[123] Atal S, Fatima Z. IL-6 inhibitors in the treatment of serious COVID-19: a promising therapy? Pharmaceut Med 2020; 34(4): 223-31.
[http://dx.doi.org/10.1007/s40290-020-00342-z] [PMID: 32535732]

[124] Michot JM, Albiges L, Chaput N, *et al.* Tocilizumab, an anti-IL-6 receptor antibody, to treat COVID-19-related respiratory failure: a case report. Ann Oncol 2020; 31(7): 961-4.
[http://dx.doi.org/10.1016/j.annonc.2020.03.300] [PMID: 32247642]

[125] Maeshima A, Nakasatomi M, Henmi D, *et al.* Efficacy of tocilizumab, a humanized neutralizing antibody against interleukin-6 receptor, in progressive renal injury associated with Castleman's disease. CEN Case Rep 2012; 1(1): 7-11.
[http://dx.doi.org/10.1007/s13730-012-0004-7] [PMID: 28509146]

[126] Filocamo G, Mangioni D, Tagliabue P, *et al.* Use of anakinra in severe COVID-19: A case report. Int J Infect Dis 2020; 96: 607-9.
[http://dx.doi.org/10.1016/j.ijid.2020.05.026] [PMID: 32437934]

[127] Cavalli G, De Luca G, Campochiaro C, *et al.* Interleukin-1 blockade with high-dose anakinra in patients with COVID-19, acute respiratory distress syndrome, and hyperinflammation: a retrospective cohort study. Lancet Rheumatol 2020; 2(6): e325-31.
[http://dx.doi.org/10.1016/S2665-9913(20)30127-2] [PMID: 32501454]

[128] USFDA. 2020 Interleukin-1 inhibitors. Silver Spring, MD: USFDA.

[129] Garfield B, Krahl T, Appel S, Cooper S, Rincón M. Regulation of p38 MAP kinase in CD4 lymphocytes by infliximab therapy in patients with rheumatoid arthritis. Clin Immunol 2005; 116(2): 101-7.
[http://dx.doi.org/10.1016/j.clim.2005.04.010] [PMID: 15914087]

[130] Hamad KM, Sabry MM, Elgayed SH, El Shabrawy AR, El-Fishawy AM, Abdel Jaleel GA. Anti-inflammatory and phytochemical evaluation of Combretum aculeatum Vent growing in Sudan. J Ethnopharmacol 2019; 242: 112052.
[http://dx.doi.org/10.1016/j.jep.2019.112052] [PMID: 31265886]

[131] Amici C, Caro AD, Ciucci A, *et al.* Indomethacin has a potent antiviral activity against SARS coronavirus. Antivir Ther 2006; 11(8): 1021-30.
[http://dx.doi.org/10.1177/135965350601100803] [PMID: 17302372]

[132] Xu T, Gao X, Wu Z, Selinger DW, Zhou Z. Indomethacin has a potent antiviral activity against SARS CoV-2 *in vitro* and canine coronavirus *in vivo*, pp. 01.017624 BioRxiv 2020; 2020; 017624.

[133] Amici C, La Frazia S, Brunelli C, Balsamo M, Angelini M, Santoro MG. Inhibition of viral protein translation by indomethacin in vesicular stomatitis virus infection: role of eIF2α kinase PKR. Cell Microbiol 2015; 17(9): 1391-404.
[http://dx.doi.org/10.1111/cmi.12446] [PMID: 25856684]

[134] Gentile LB, Queiroz-Hazarbassanov N, Massoco CO, Fecchio D. Modulation of cytokines production by indomethacin acute dose during the evolution of Ehrlich ascites tumor in Mice. Mediators Inflamm 2015; 2015: 1-8.
[http://dx.doi.org/10.1155/2015/924028] [PMID: 26347589]

[135] Shacter E, Arzadon GK, Williams J. Elevation of interleukin-6 in response to a chronic inflammatory stimulus in mice: inhibition by indomethacin. Blood 1992; 80(1): 194-202.
[http://dx.doi.org/10.1182/blood.V80.1.194.194] [PMID: 1611085]

[136] Zhou W, Liu Y, Tian D, *et al.* Potential benefits of precise corticosteroids therapy for severe 2019-nCoV pneumonia. Signal Transduct Target Ther 2020; 5(1): 18.
[http://dx.doi.org/10.1038/s41392-020-0127-9] [PMID: 32296012]

[137] Paravar T, Lee DJ. Thalidomide: Mechanisms of Action. Int Rev Immunol 2008; 27(3): 111-35.
[http://dx.doi.org/10.1080/08830180801911339] [PMID: 18437602]

[138] Albuquerque D, Nihei J, Cardillo F, Singh R. The ACE inhibitors enalapril and captopril modulate cytokine responses in Balb/c and C57Bl/6 normal mice and increase CD4+CD103+CD25negative splenic T cell numbers. Cell Immunol 2010; 260(2): 92-7.
[http://dx.doi.org/10.1016/j.cellimm.2009.09.006] [PMID: 19854435]

[139] Lee C, Chun J, Hwang SW, Kang SJ, Im JP, Kim JS. Enalapril inhibits nuclear factor-κB signaling in intestinal epithelial cells and peritoneal macrophages and attenuates experimental colitis in mice. Life Sci 2014; 95(1): 29-39.
[http://dx.doi.org/10.1016/j.lfs.2013.11.005] [PMID. 24239644]

[140] Choe SH, Choi EY, Hyeon JY, Keum BR, Choi IS, Kim SJ. Telmisartan, an angiotensin II receptor blocker, attenuates Prevotella intermedia lipopolysaccharide-induced production of nitric oxide and interleukin-1β in murine macrophages. Int Immunopharmacol 2019; 75: 105750.
[http://dx.doi.org/10.1016/j.intimp.2019.105750] [PMID: 31330445]

[141] Saber S, Basuony M, Eldin AS. Telmisartan ameliorates dextran sodium sulfate-induced colitis in rats by modulating NF-κB signalling in the context of PPARγ agonistic activity. Arch Biochem Biophys 2019; 671: 185-95.
[http://dx.doi.org/10.1016/j.abb.2019.07.014] [PMID: 31326516]

[142] Gurwitz D. Angiotensin receptor blockers as tentative SARS-CoV-2 therapeutics. Drug Dev Res 2020; 81(5): 537-40.
[http://dx.doi.org/10.1002/ddr.21656] [PMID: 32129518]

[143] Ishiyama Y, Gallagher PE, Averill DB, Tallant EA, Brosnihan KB, Ferrario CM. Upregulation of angiotensin-converting enzyme 2 after myocardial infarction by blockade of angiotensin II receptors. Hypertension 2004; 43(5): 970-6.
[http://dx.doi.org/10.1161/01.HYP.0000124667.34652.1a] [PMID: 15007027]

[144] Rukavina Mikusic NL, Kouyoumdzian NM, Uceda A, et al. Losartan prevents the imbalance between renal dopaminergic and renin angiotensin systems induced by fructose overload. l-Dopa/dopamine index as new potential biomarker of renal dysfunction. Metabolism 2018; 85: 271-85.
[http://dx.doi.org/10.1016/j.metabol.2018.04.010] [PMID: 29727629]

[145] Wang X, Chen X, Huang W, et al. Losartan suppresses the inflammatory response in collagen-induced arthritis by inhibiting the MAPK and NF-κB pathways in B and T cells. Inflammopharmacology 2019; 27(3): 487-502.
[http://dx.doi.org/10.1007/s10787-018-0545-2] [PMID: 30426454]

[146] Ajayi S, Becker H, Reinhardt H, et al. Ruxolitinib InSmall molecules in Hematology 2018; 119-32.
[http://dx.doi.org/10.1007/978-3-319-91439-8_6]

[147] Treon SP, Castillo JJ, Skarbnik AP, et al. The BTK inhibitor ibrutinib may protect against pulmonary injury in COVID-19–infected patients. Blood 2020; 135(21): 1912-5.
[http://dx.doi.org/10.1182/blood.2020006288] [PMID: 32302379]

[148] Einhaus J, Pecher AC, Asteriti E, et al. Inhibition of effector B cells by ibrutinib in systemic sclerosis. Arthritis Res Ther 2020; 22(1): 66.
[http://dx.doi.org/10.1186/s13075-020-02153-8] [PMID: 32228672]

[149] González Canga A, Sahagún Prieto AM, Diez Liébana MJ, Fernández Martínez N, Sierra Vega M, García Vieitez JJ. The pharmacokinetics and interactions of ivermectin in humans--a mini-review. AAPS J 2008; 10(1): 42-6.
[http://dx.doi.org/10.1208/s12248-007-9000-9] [PMID: 18446504]

[150] Caly L, Druce JD, Catton MG, Jans DA, Wagstaff KM. The FDA-approved drug ivermectin inhibits the replication of SARS-CoV-2 in vitro. Antiviral Res 2020; 178: 104787.
[http://dx.doi.org/10.1016/j.antiviral.2020.104787] [PMID: 32251768]

[151] Lv C, Liu W, Wang B, et al. Ivermectin inhibits DNA polymerase UL42 of pseudorabies virus entrance into the nucleus and proliferation of the virus in vitro and vivo. Antiviral Res 2018; 159: 55-62.
[http://dx.doi.org/10.1016/j.antiviral.2018.09.010] [PMID: 30266338]

[152] Tay MYF, Fraser JE, Chan WKK, et al. Nuclear localization of dengue virus (DENV) 1–4 non-structural protein 5; protection against all 4 DENV serotypes by the inhibitor Ivermectin. Antiviral Res

2013; 99(3): 301-6.
[http://dx.doi.org/10.1016/j.antiviral.2013.06.002] [PMID: 23769930]

[153] Crump A. Ivermectin: enigmatic multifaceted 'wonder' drug continues to surprise and exceed expectations. J Antibiot (Tokyo) 2017; 70(5): 495-505.
[http://dx.doi.org/10.1038/ja.2017.11] [PMID: 28196978]

[154] Sajid MS, Iqbal Z, Muhammad G, Iqbal MU. Immunomodulatory effect of various anti-parasitics: a review. Parasitology 2006; 132(3): 301-13.
[http://dx.doi.org/10.1017/S0031182005009108] [PMID: 16332285]

[155] Yan S, Ci X, Chen N, *et al*. Anti-inflammatory effects of ivermectin in mouse model of allergic asthma. Inflamm Res 2011; 60(6): 589-96.
[http://dx.doi.org/10.1007/s00011-011-0307-8] [PMID: 21279416]

[156] Zhang X, Song Y, Ci X, *et al*. Ivermectin inhibits LPS-induced production of inflammatory cytokines and improves LPS-induced survival in mice. Inflamm Res 2008; 57(11): 524-9.
[http://dx.doi.org/10.1007/s00011-008-8007-8] [PMID: 19109745]

[157] PAHO/WHO, COVID-19: Chloroquine and hydroxychloroquine research. 2020.
https:iris.paho.org/handle/10665.2/52105

[158] Yao X, Ye F, Zhang M, *et al*. *In vitro* antiviral activity and projection of optimized dosing design of hydroxychloroquine for the treatment of severe acute respiratory syndrome coronavirus 2 (SARS-CoV-2). Clin Infect Dis 2020; 71(15): 732-9.
[http://dx.doi.org/10.1093/cid/ciaa237] [PMID: 32150618]

[159] Rösler B, Herold S. Lung epithelial GM-CSF improves host defense function and epithelial repair in influenza virus pneumonia—a new therapeutic strategy? Mol Cell Pediatr 2016; 3(1): 29.
[http://dx.doi.org/10.1186/s40348-016-0055-5] [PMID: 27480877]

[160] Paine R III, Wilcoxen SE, Morris SB, *et al*. Transgenic overexpression of granulocyte macrophage-colony stimulating factor in the lung prevents hyperoxic lung injury. Am J Pathol 2003; 163(6): 2397-406.
[http://dx.doi.org/10.1016/S0002-9440(10)63594-8] [PMID: 14633611]

[161] Baleeiro CEO, Christensen PJ, Morris SB, Mendez MP, Wilcoxen SE, Paine R III. GM-CSF and the impaired pulmonary innate immune response following hyperoxic stress. Am J Physiol Lung Cell Mol Physiol 2006; 291(6): L1246-55.
[http://dx.doi.org/10.1152/ajplung.00016.2006] [PMID: 16891399]

[162] Matute-Bello G, Liles CW, Radella F II, *et al*. Modulation of neutrophil apoptosis by granulocyte colony-stimulating factor and granulocyte/macrophage colony-stimulating factor during the course of acute respiratory distress syndrome. Crit Care Med 2000; 28(1): 1-7.
[http://dx.doi.org/10.1097/00003246-200001000-00001] [PMID: 10667491]

[163] Talotta R. Do COVID-19 RNA-based vaccines put at risk of immune-mediated diseases? In reply to "potential antigenic cross-reactivity between SARS-CoV-2 and human tissue with a possible link to an increase in autoimmune diseases". Clin Immunol 2021; 224: 108665.
[http://dx.doi.org/10.1016/j.clim.2021.108665] [PMID: 33429060]

[164] Martínez GJ, Robertson S, Barraclough J, *et al*. Colchicine acutely suppresses local cardiac production of inflammatory cytokines in patients with an acute coronary syndrome. J Am Heart Assoc 2015; 4(8): e002128.
[http://dx.doi.org/10.1161/JAHA.115.002128] [PMID: 26304941]

[165] Leung YY, Hui LL, Kraus VB. Colchicine—update on mechanisms of action and therapeutic uses. InSeminars in arthritis and rheumatism 2015 Dec 1 (Vol. 45, No. 3, pp. 341-350). WB Saunders.

[166] Cumhur Cure M, Kucuk A, Cure E. Colchicine may not be effective in COVID-19 infection; it may even be harmful? Clin Rheumatol 2020; 39(7): 2101-2.
[http://dx.doi.org/10.1007/s10067-020-05144-x] [PMID: 32394215]

[167] Gendelman O, Amital H, Bragazzi NL, Watad A, Chodick G. Continuous hydroxychloroquine or colchicine therapy does not prevent infection with SARS-CoV-2: Insights from a large healthcare database analysis. Autoimmun Rev 2020; 19(7): 102566.
[http://dx.doi.org/10.1016/j.autrev.2020.102566] [PMID: 32380315]

[168] Klok FA, Kruip MJHA, van der Meer NJM, *et al.* Incidence of thrombotic complications in critically ill ICU patients with COVID-19. Thromb Res 2020; 191: 145-7.
[http://dx.doi.org/10.1016/j.thromres.2020.04.013] [PMID: 32291094]

[169] Middeldorp S, Coppens M, Haaps TF, *et al.* Incidence of venous thromboembolism in hospitalized patients with COVID 19. J Thromb Haemost 2020; 18(8): 1995-2002.
[http://dx.doi.org/10.1111/jth.14888] [PMID: 32369666]

[170] Moores LK, Tritschler T, Brosnahan S, *et al.* Prevention, diagnosis, and treatment of VTe in patients with coronavirus disease 2019. Chest 2020; 158(3): 1143-63.
[http://dx.doi.org/10.1016/j.chest.2020.05.559] [PMID: 32502594]

[171] Giannis D, Ziogas IA, Gianni P. Coagulation disorders in coronavirus infected patients: COVID-19, SARS-CoV-1, MERS-CoV and lessons from the past. J Clin Virol 2020; 127: 104362.
[http://dx.doi.org/10.1016/j.jcv.2020.104362] [PMID: 32305883]

[172] Obi AT, Tignanelli CJ, Jacobs BN, *et al.* Empirical systemic anticoagulation is associated with decreased venous thromboembolism in critically ill influenza A H1N1 acute respiratory distress syndrome patients. J Vasc Surg Venous Lymphat Disord 2019; 7(3): 317-24.
[http://dx.doi.org/10.1016/j.jvsv.2018.08.010] [PMID: 30477976]

[173] Helms J, Tacquard C, Severac F, *et al.* High risk of thrombosis in patients with severe SARS-CoV-2 infection: a multicenter prospective cohort study. Intensive Care Med 2020; 46(6): 1089-98.
[http://dx.doi.org/10.1007/s00134-020-06062-x] [PMID: 32367170]

[174] Llitjos JF, Leclerc M, Chochois C, *et al.* High incidence of venous thromboembolic events in anticoagulated severe COVID 19 patients. J Thromb Haemost 2020; 18(7): 1743-6.
[http://dx.doi.org/10.1111/jth.14869] [PMID: 32320517]

[175] Desborough MJR, Doyle AJ, Griffiths A, Retter A, Breen KA, Hunt BJ. Image-proven thromboembolism in patients with severe COVID-19 in a tertiary critical care unit in the United Kingdom. Thromb Res 2020; 193: 1-4.
[http://dx.doi.org/10.1016/j.thromres.2020.05.049] [PMID: 32485437]

[176] Engelmann B, Massberg S. Thrombosis as an intravascular effector of innate immunity. Nat Rev Immunol 2013; 13(1): 34-45.
[http://dx.doi.org/10.1038/nri3345] [PMID: 23222502]

[177] Loo J, Spittle DA, Newnham M. COVID-19, immunothrombosis and venous thromboembolism: biological mechanisms. Thorax 2021; 76(4): 412-20.
[http://dx.doi.org/10.1136/thoraxjnl-2020-216243] [PMID: 33408195]

[178] Rico-Mesa JS, Rosas D, Ahmadian-Tehrani A, White A, Anderson AS, Chilton R. The role of anticoagulation in COVID-19-induced hypercoagulability. Curr Cardiol Rep 2020; 22(7): 53.
[http://dx.doi.org/10.1007/s11886-020-01328-8] [PMID: 32556892]

[179] Zhang Y, Xiao M, Zhang S, *et al.* Coagulopathy and antiphospholipid antibodies in patients with Covid-19. N Engl J Med 2020; 382(17): e38.
[http://dx.doi.org/10.1056/NEJMc2007575] [PMID: 32268022]

[180] Uthman IW, Gharavi AE. Viral infections and antiphospholipid antibodies. Seminars in arthritis and rheumatism. WB Saunders 2002; 31: pp. (4)256-63.
[http://dx.doi.org/10.1053/sarh.2002.28303]

[181] Li T, Lu H, Zhang W. Clinical observation and management of COVID-19 patients. Emerg Microbes Infect 2020; 9(1): 687-90.
[http://dx.doi.org/10.1080/22221751.2020.1741327] [PMID: 32208840]

[182]   Wright FL, Vogler TO, Moore EE, *et al.* Fibrinolysis shutdown correlation with thromboembolic events in severe COVID-19 infection. J Am Coll Surg 2020; 231(2): 193-203e1.
[http://dx.doi.org/10.1016/j.jamcollsurg.2020.05.007] [PMID: 32422349]

[183]   Bao J, Li C, Zhang K, Kang H, Chen W, Gu B. Comparative analysis of laboratory indexes of severe and non-severe patients infected with COVID-19. Clin Chim Acta 2020; 509: 180-94.
[http://dx.doi.org/10.1016/j.cca.2020.06.009] [PMID: 32511971]

[184]   Iba T, Levy JH, Connors JM, Warkentin TE, Thachil J, Levi M. The unique characteristics of COVID-19 coagulopathy. Crit Care 2020; 24(1): 360.
[http://dx.doi.org/10.1186/s13054-020-03077-0] [PMID: 32552865]

[185]   Olson JD. D-dimer. Adv Clin Chem 2015; 69: 1-46.
[http://dx.doi.org/10.1016/bs.acc.2014.12.001] [PMID: 25934358]

[186]   Tang N, Bai H, Chen X, Gong J, Li D, Sun Z. Anticoagulant treatment is associated with decreased mortality in severe coronavirus disease 2019 patients with coagulopathy. J Thromb Haemost 2020; 18(5): 1094-9.
[http://dx.doi.org/10.1111/jth.14817] [PMID: 32220112]

[187]   Cummings MJ, Baldwin MR, Abrams D, *et al.* Epidemiology, clinical course, and outcomes of critically ill adults with COVID-19 in New York City: a prospective cohort study. Lancet 2020; 395(10239): 1763-70.
[http://dx.doi.org/10.1016/S0140-6736(20)31189-2] [PMID: 32442528]

[188]   Yau JW, Teoh H, Verma S. Endothelial cell control of thrombosis. BMC Cardiovasc Disord 2015; 15(1): 130.
[http://dx.doi.org/10.1186/s12872-015-0124-z] [PMID: 26481314]

[189]   Hadi HA, Carr CS, Al Suwaidi J. Endothelial dysfunction: cardiovascular risk factors, therapy, and outcome. Vasc Health Risk Manag 2005; 1(3): 183-98.
[PMID: 17319104]

[190]   Ackermann M, Verleden SE, Kuehnel M, *et al.* Pulmonary vascular endothelialitis, thrombosis, and angiogenesis in Covid-19. N Engl J Med 2020; 383(2): 120-8.
[http://dx.doi.org/10.1056/NEJMoa2015432] [PMID: 32437596]

[191]   Huertas A, Montani D, Savale L, *et al.* Endothelial cell dysfunction: a major player in SARS-CoV-2 infection (COVID-19)? Eur Respir J 2020; 56(1): 2001634.
[http://dx.doi.org/10.1183/13993003.01634-2020] [PMID: 32554538]

[192]   Hoffmann M, Kleine-Weber H, Schroeder S, *et al.* SARS-CoV-2 cell entry depends on ACE2 and TMPRSS2 and is blocked by a clinically proven protease inhibitor. Cell 2020; 181(2): 271-280.e8.
[http://dx.doi.org/10.1016/j.cell.2020.02.052] [PMID: 32142651]

[193]   Tay MZ, Poh CM, Rénia L, MacAry PA, Ng LFP. The trinity of COVID-19: immunity, inflammation and intervention. Nat Rev Immunol 2020; 20(6): 363-74.
[http://dx.doi.org/10.1038/s41577-020-0311-8] [PMID: 32346093]

[194]   Connors JM, Levy JH. COVID-19 and its implications for thrombosis and anticoagulation. Blood 2020; 135(23): 2033-40.
[http://dx.doi.org/10.1182/blood.2020006000] [PMID: 32339221]

[195]   Ellinghaus D, Degenhardt F, Bujanda L, *et al.* Genomewide association study of severe Covid-19 with respiratory failure. N Engl J Med 2020; 383(16): 1522-34.
[http://dx.doi.org/10.1056/NEJMoa2020283] [PMID: 32558485]

[196]   Bikdeli B, Madhavan MV, Jimenez D, *et al.* COVID-19 and thrombotic or thromboembolic disease: implications for prevention, antithrombotic therapy, and follow-up: JACC state-of-the-art review. J Am Coll Cardiol 2020; 75(23): 2950-73.
[http://dx.doi.org/10.1016/j.jacc.2020.04.031] [PMID: 32311448]

[197] Pannucci CJ, Fleming KI, Holoyda K, Moulton L, Prazak AM, Varghese TK Jr. Enoxaparin 40 mg per day is inadequate for venous thromboembolism prophylaxis after thoracic surgical procedure. Ann Thorac Surg 2018; 106(2): 404-11.
[http://dx.doi.org/10.1016/j.athoracsur.2018.02.085] [PMID: 29626461]

[198] Wang TF, Milligan PE, Wong CA, Deal EN, Thoelke MS, Gage BF. Efficacy and safety of high-dose thromboprophylaxis in morbidly obese inpatients. Thromb Haemost 2014; 111(1): 88-93.
[http://dx.doi.org/10.1160/TH13-01-0042] [PMID: 24136071]

[199] Ranucci M, Ballotta A, Di Dedda U, *et al.* The procoagulant pattern of patients with COVID-19 acute respiratory distress syndrome. J Thromb Haemost 2020; 18(7): 1747-51.
[http://dx.doi.org/10.1111/jth.14854] [PMID: 32302448]

[200] Tang N, Li D, Wang X, Sun Z. Abnormal coagulation parameters are associated with poor prognosis in patients with novel coronavirus pneumonia. J Thromb Haemost 2020; 18(4): 844-7.
[http://dx.doi.org/10.1111/jth.14768] [PMID: 32073213]

[201] Vicenzi E, Canducci F, Pinna D, *et al.* Coronaviridae and SARS-associated coronavirus strain HSR1. Emerg Infect Dis 2004; 10(3): 413-8.
[http://dx.doi.org/10.3201/eid1003.030683] [PMID: 15109406]

[202] Du L, Kao RY, Zhou Y, *et al.* Cleavage of spike protein of SARS coronavirus by protease factor Xa is associated with viral infectivity. Biochem Biophys Res Commun 2007; 359(1): 174-9.
[http://dx.doi.org/10.1016/j.bbrc.2007.05.092] [PMID: 17533109]

[203] Kam YW, Okumura Y, Kido H, Ng LFP, Bruzzone R, Altmeyer R. Cleavage of the SARS coronavirus spike glycoprotein by airway proteases enhances virus entry into human bronchial epithelial cells *in vitro*. PLoS One 2009; 4(11): e7870.
[http://dx.doi.org/10.1371/journal.pone.0007870] [PMID: 19924243]

[204] Smyth SS, McEver RP, Weyrich AS, *et al.* Platelet functions beyond hemostasis. J Thromb Haemost 2009; 7(11): 1759-66.
[http://dx.doi.org/10.1111/j.1538-7836.2009.03586.x] [PMID: 19691483]

CHAPTER 6

High Throughput Screening (HTS) Methods for Screening of Known Drugs for COVID-19

Tejal Shreeya[1,2] and **Tabish Qidwai**[3,*]

[1] *Institute of Biophysics, Biological Research Centre, Szeged, Hungary, Europe*

[2] *Doctoral School of Theoretical Medicine, University of Szeged, Hungary, Europe*

[3] *Faculty of Biotechnology, Shriramswaroop Memorial University, Lucknow, UP, India*

Abstract: The emergence of severe acute respiratory syndrome coronavirus 2 (SARS-CoV-2) in late 2019 has triggered an ongoing global pandemic whereby infection may result in a lethal severe pneumonia-like disease designated as coronavirus disease 2019 (COVID-19). Thus, the repositioning of known drugs can significantly accelerate the development and deployment of therapies for COVID-19.

High throughput screening (HTS) is the use of automated equipment to rapidly test thousands to millions of samples for biological activity at the model organism, cellular, pathway, or molecular level. In its most common form, HTS is an experimental process in which 10^3–10^6 small molecule compounds of known structure are screened in parallel. Currently, this technique is being used to screen known compounds in several diseases, including COVID-19. In the current scenario, it is important to focus on the application of high-throughput screening (HTS) in the drug discovery process.

In this chapter, we have covered methods of the high-throughput screen and its use in screening known drugs against infectious diseases like COVID-19. Moreover, the challenges and future of these technologies have been focussed.

Keywords: COVID-19, Drug discovery, High Throughput Screening, SARS-CoV-2.

INTRODUCTION

A clinical condition or a disease in the body leads to the initiation of drug discovery. The unmet clinical need provokes the discovery of the drug. The process of drug discovery starts with a 'hypothesis' that is the result of initial research. The hypothesis may include activation or inhibition of any protein, enz-

---

* **Corresponding author Tabish Qidwai**: Faculty of Biotechnology, Shriramswaroop Memorial University, Lucknow, UP, India; E-mail: tabish.iet@gmail.com

yme, or metabolic pathway. The hypothesis later resulted in a therapeutic effect in a disease state [1]. Drug discovery is a highly complex, tedious and multidisciplinary process, and its ultimate goal is to recognize new drugs with desired characteristics. A single marketed drug emerges from approximately a million screened compounds. For this, large compound libraries are screened. The process of drug discovery starts with the identification of suitable drug targets, which includes molecules such as enzymes and receptors, at times, ion channels also. Enzymes such as kinases, phosphatases, proteases and peptidases are the most common targets of HTS [2]. The next step is the target validation which is done *in vitro* and *in vivo* on animals. The ultimate validation is achieved in humans. Fig. (**1**) shows the entire process of Drug discovery. The modulators may be in respect to the target, such as agonist or antagonist, while in the case of receptors, it may be an activator or an inhibitor [3].

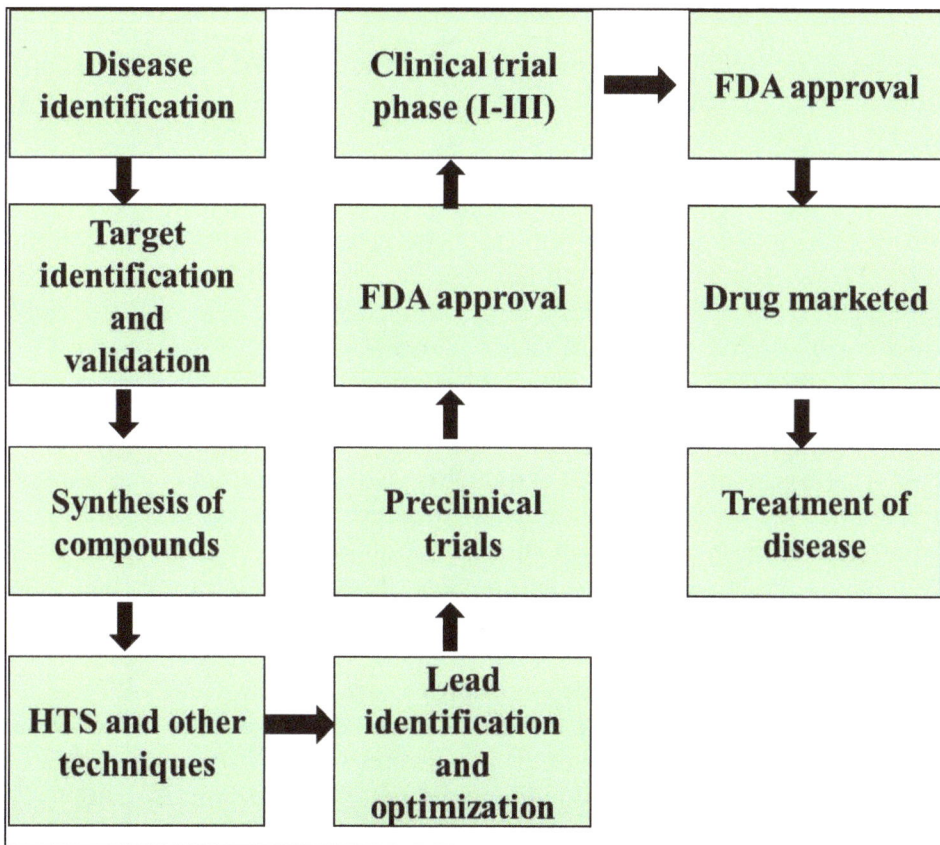

Fig. (1). Flowchart showing the process of drug discovery.

Hit identification and lead optimization are very much intertwined with computational modelling [4]. The ultimate goal of target validation leads to "lead identification". For the purpose of target validation, various suitable assays are designed and developed. HTS exposes the target to various compound libraries in order to get lead identification. The selection of lead identification depends on selectivity, pharmacokinetics and physicochemical properties [3].

High Throughput Screening

High throughput screening is one of the most important method for the discovery of drugs in this modern technological world. It is used to identify "hits" from known compound libraries that might become a "lead" compound for optimization of the drug in the future. HTS is the first step in the search for an active compound with the potential to develop into an active compound.

This technology relies on various other branches of science, such as bioinformatics, combinatorial chemistry and parallel synthesis approaches. The ability to test a huge number of compounds quickly and efficiently provides a competitive opportunity, making HTS a crucial tool in many pharmaceutical companies which exploits this technique for the discovery of the drug [5]. Bioinformatics, genomics and proteomics help in the identification of novel biological targets that are related to the disease. The parallel synthesis approach and combinational chemistry yields a large number of small compounds which are already available for the purpose of drug discovery.

The primary purpose of screening is to search the compound libraries and recognize a compound that has desired characteristics and could interact with the selected system in a proper way. For this purpose various compounds are being assayed against the target in order to get a specific mechanism of action for *e.g.*, in the case of an enzyme, its activation or inhibition by the compound or its receptor-ligand interaction. The compound of interest with all the desired activities is recognized and is then allowed to undergo different biological assays in order to optimize the efficacy and drug-like properties. The refinement/processing of the compound properties is known as "hit" to "lead" process. The ultimate goal of the screening is to develop a drug candidate with desired characteristics which could be further used for optimization and development of a new drug useful in the treatment of the disease [6]. The inverted pyramid in Fig. (**2**) shows how the ultimate compound of interest is achieved.

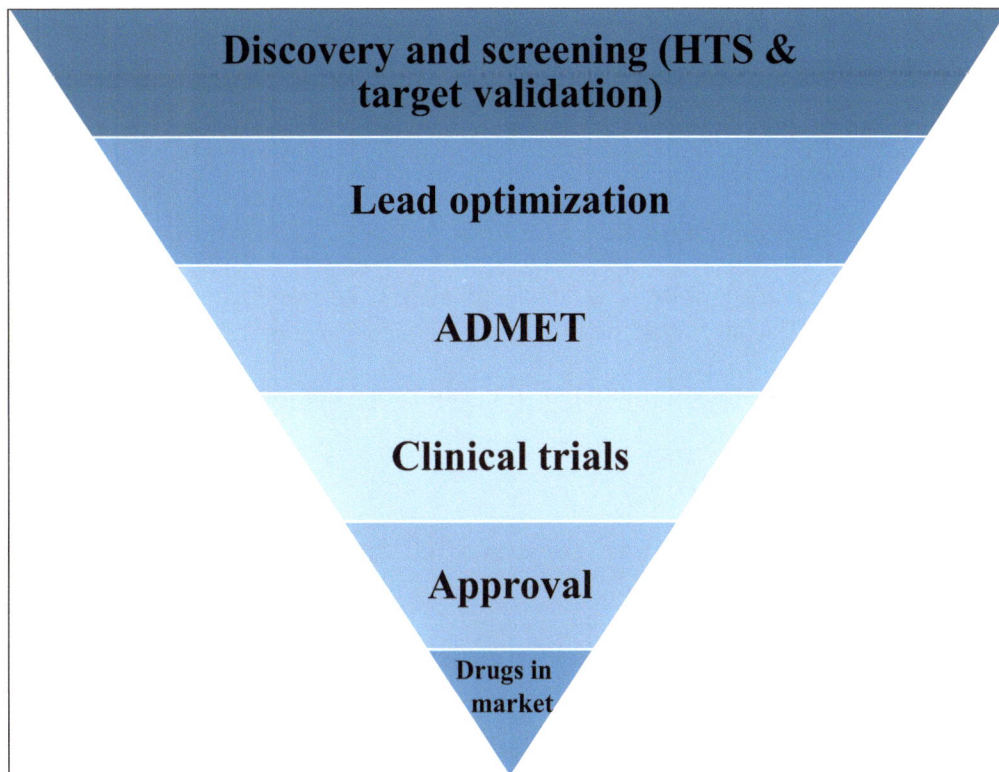

Fig. (2). Inverted pyramid showing the number of compounds selected initially are too large, while at every step lot of compounds are rejected, and finally a single compound is selected with desired characteristics is marketed in the form of the drug.

The HTS was developed in the year 1986 [7]. Before 1986, screening was performed manually, which was time-consuming, and the identification of "hits" was a challenging thing. The technique used was receptor binding assay. With the development of automated devices and laboratory robots, no. of compounds being screened has gradually increased per unit of time and also reduced time consumption. In the modern era, the HTS is now replaced by ultra HTS (uHTS), in which more than 100,000 compounds are being screened against a single target per unit time. Pharmaceutical companies are the one who utilizes the HTS as the major component of drug discovery.

Compound Library

In order to identify new hits, large compound libraries are screened. The compound library store information on hundreds of thousand of compounds. They are differentiated into various groups and subgroups on the basis of their size, structure and chemical and physical properties which provides an easy platform for the search of the initial "hit" compound. Dividing them into groups and subgroups reduces time and is also cost-effective. In the case of a "novel target" about which nothing is known, random libraries with diverse "drug-like" structures are used [8].

Some of the compound libraries are as follows:

1. FDA approved drug library- consists of all the compounds that are already approved by the FDA and other health agencies.

2. Inhibitor related library-contains all the inhibitory compounds such as kinase, protease

3. Diversity compound library.

4. Natural product and medicine- consists of all the natural products as well as alkaloids and flavonoids.

5. Neuronal and immunologically related- consists of neuronal and immune-related compounds.

6. Metabolism related- consists of all the compounds related to various metabolisms such as glycolysis, lipid metabolism, gut microbial compound, *etc.*

7. By Signalling pathway- consists of compounds related to the signalling pathways. It is further divided into different signalling pathway compounds.

8. By disease- compounds are present according to various diseases

9. Bioactive compound library- consists of a unique collection of bioactive compounds.

10. Epigenomic library-

11. Cell death library- consists of compounds related to cell death, such as apoptosis and autophagy.

12. Anti-infective library- consists of compounds that are anti-infectious.

13. NCATS pharmaceutical collection (NPC)-consists of ~3000 drugs, which are FDA-approved and also approved by some other health agencies in Europe and other countries.

14. MIPE (Mechanism Interrogation Plate)- Bioactive compounds that target mechanism of action

15. NPACT (NCATS pharmacologically active chemical toolbox)- contains mechanistically defined molecules and natural products.

Methods of HTS

With the development of science and new technologies, the process of HTS has developed with a number of assays for the optimization of the "lead" compound into a novel drug. From classical and traditional techniques to modern ones are discussed in this chapter.

Biochemical Assays

These assays measure the ligand interaction and enzymatic inhibition and work competitively as the compound of interest must displace a known ligand or substrate (Fig. **3**).

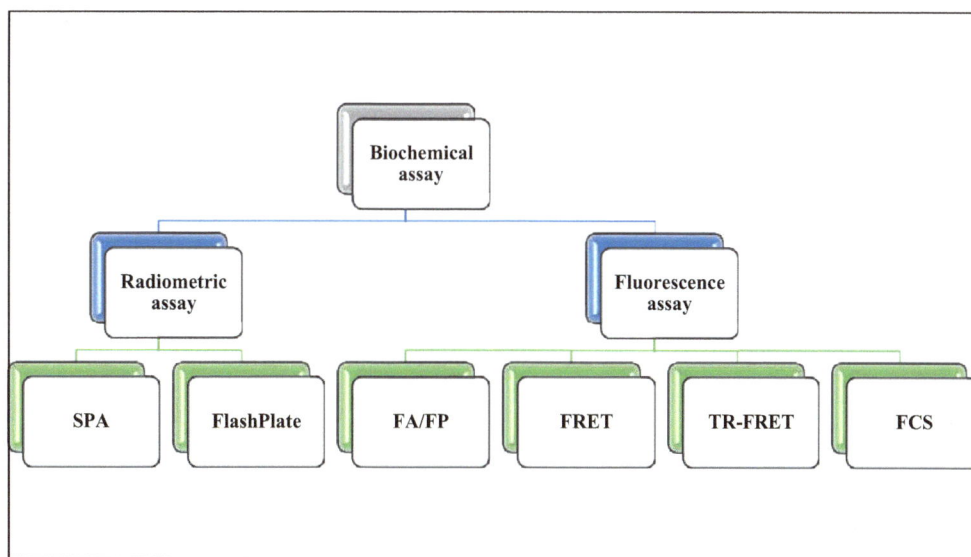

Fig. (3). Flowchart showing the Biochemical assays.

Radiometric Assays

The radiometric assay is one the oldest assays introduced in the 90's. Since then, a lot of advancement has taken place. It constitutes 20-50% of all the screenings performed. Its use has now decreased, and with time, it shall completely disappear.

SPA (Scintillating Proximity Assay)

In this assay, the acceptor molecules are already immobilized in the scintillating beads, and the ligand is radioactive. When this radioactive ligand binds to the acceptor attached to the scintillating bead, the radiation is converted into light, which could be easily quantified. The quantity of light emitted is proportional to the quantity of radio-ligand bound, while the free radio-ligand remains undetected. SPA is generally suitable for receptor-ligand binding assays, but protein-protein interaction, immunoassays, and other enzyme assays are also suitable [5]. Fig. (**4A**) is a diagrammatical representation of SPA.

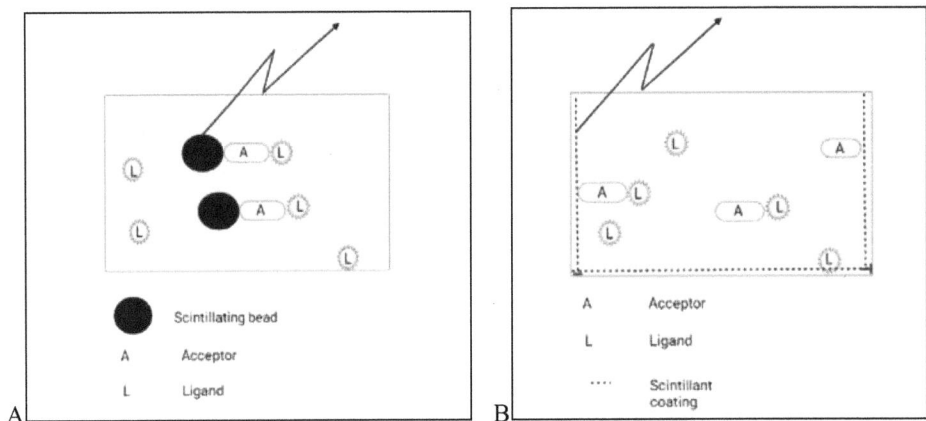

Fig. (4). (A) showing the SPA in which the acceptor is attached to the scintillating bead while **(B)** shows FlashPlate assay in which the acceptor is attached to the scintillant coated plate.

FlashPlate Assay

It is very much similar to the SPA assay. The only difference is that instead of the scintillating beads, the plate is scintillant coated. The ligand binds to the acceptor attached the scintillant-coated plate. Diagrammatic representation is shown in Fig. (**4B**).

The classical approach of the HTS exploits the conventional receptor binding and enzymology protocol. The enzymatic assays utilize the chemically modified substrate that somehow leads to a change in fluorescence which is used for optimization. The major drawback of radioactive technique is the sensitivity and readout times f detection instruments.

Fluorescence assays have an advantage over radioactive ones, majorly being safety issues. They have higher sensitivity in comparison to the radioactive assays, are easy to handle and can be easily miniaturized, which was again a major drawback of the radioactive assays.

Fluorescence Assays

Fluorescence polarization (FP), Fluorescence resonance energy transfer (FRET) and fluorescence correlation spectroscopy (FCS) are the traditional fluorescence methods used in HTS. They are mostly used to study molecular interaction.

Fluorescence Anisotropy and Fluorescence Polarization (FA/FP)

Fluorescence polarization and anisotropy go hand in hand, which means they are nearly equivalent techniques used in HTS in drug discovery. This assay is fast, sensitive, resistant to some interferences, and inexpensive [9]. It yields information about molecular rotations in events such as receptor-ligand binding and enzymatic assays. It can be used with various biochemical strategies in efficient screens.

FP assays report changes in molecular weight. This assay is exploited to interrogate various biological processes involving protein-protein, protein-peptide interactions and enzymatic activity as well. In FP, when fluorescence molecules are excited by polarized light in one plane, the emitted fluorescent signal also becomes plane polarized. The alteration in molecular weight of the fluorescent probe or the tracer is indicated by changes in the polarization of sample's emitted light [10].

Fluorescence Resonance Energy Transfer (FRET)

FRET is also known as Forster resonance energy transfer. FRET was described by Morrison in the year 1988. It is the result of fluorescence transfer between acceptor and donor fluorochromes *via* dipole-dipole interaction. FRET occurs only if there is compatibility between the excitable and emission wavelengths. The acceptor molecule is transferred to a higher level, and while returning to the ground state, it emits fluorescent light, which is recorded. The efficiency of energy transfer depends on spectral overlap between donor and acceptor, their distance and relative orientation. The substrate is phosphorylated in order to bring the donor and the acceptor in close proximity so that the FRET could occur. Organic molecules like fluorescein or rhodamine-conjugated to protein pair or fluorescent proteins fused to a protein of interest are used as dyes. The other fluorophores used in FRET are mutant GFPs (Green Fluorescent Proteins), and cyanine fluorochromes [5, 11].

Time Resolves Fluorescence Resonance Energy Transfer (TR-FRET)

TR-FRET is the variant of FRET and is widely used in screening. It is based on long-range energy transfer between fluorescence Lanthanide complexes (Ln^{+3}) as donors and an acceptor with suitable resonance energy [3]. Lanthanide complexes, such as Europium, *etc.*, which have long wavelengths as donors along with fluorescent proteins or organic fluorophores, are used as acceptors.

The fluorophore emission of the acceptor is gated so that the emission of shorter fluorophores decays by the time signal is acquired. A time gap (Stroke shift) is set between the excitation of a fluorophore and the reading of the emission signal in order to decay all the background fluorescence and measure only the lanthanide fluorescence [6, 12].

Fluorescence Correlation Spectroscopy

It is a technique that measures molecular fluorescence fluctuation and the abundance, mobility and interaction of fluorescently labelled biomolecules [13]. The observation volume is as small as 1 femtoliter, sometimes even less than this. In this assay, the biological actions could be observed easily [6]. This technique can even screen extracellular vesicles, and cell-derived vesicles [14]. The advantage of using this FCS is that it can be used to detect the very minute volume of the sample.

Binding Based Assays

The binding-based assays are based on biophysical techniques and use small libraries compared to the biochemical assays, which use large compound libraries. These assays are used for the challenging orphan targets about which nothing is known. They are used for other drug discovery processes, such as hit validation and lead optimization. It detects membrane permeability and cytotoxicity (Fig. **5**).

Fragment-based Drug Design (FBDD)

It is suitable for biophysical methods. It is used to screen fragments of small molecules, mostly less than 280 Da. These small molecule fragments have weak interaction. This technique mostly targets protein-protein interaction and orphan targets. FBDD has an advantage over traditional HTS methods; it achieves higher hit rates, as it is among the improved assays of drug design. Some computational strategies are applied in the process of FBDD [15]. This technique has been showing increased promise in the field of drug discovery, and we hope to continue with this in the future as well. This assay uses different methods of detection such as NMR (Nuclear Magnetic Resonance), SPR (Surface Plasmon Resonance) and x-ray crystallography [16].

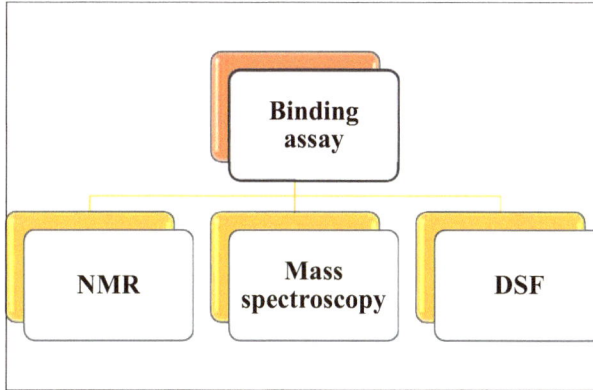

Fig. (5). Flowchart showing the Binding assays.

Cell-based Assays

It is used for compounds whose molecular targets are unknown and to screen multiple targets at once. Cell-based assays are used only when the target cannot be used in biochemical assays. Fig. (**6**) shows the flowchart of all the cell based assay. It provides information about the mechanism of action that the receptor binding assays lack. It even provides information about the membrane permeability and cytotoxicity of compounds. It is the only assay that can be used throughout the drug discovery process.

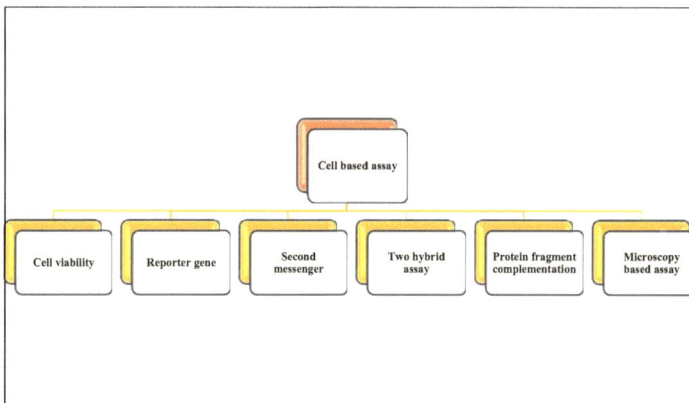

Fig. (6). Flowing the Cell based assays used in HTS.

Most commonly used approaches of cell-based assays are as follows:

• Cell viability

• Secondary messenger

• Reporter gene

• Protein fragment complementation

• Yeast two hybrid assay

• Microscopy based assays

The Cell Viability Assay

identifies compounds that kill/destroy cancer cells or pathogens. Most commonly, the ATP content is measured using the luciferase to generate the luminescence in an ATP-dependent reaction. Dyes such as ruthenium and tetrazolium are used in the viability assay. The viability or death of the assay is indicated by the change in the fluorescence.

Reporter Gene Assay

In this assay, the signalling pathway is selected, and a sequence is prepared that codes for the reporter gene. The reporter is now expressed into the transcriptional stage, and its expression is monitored *via* luminescence and fluorescence that tells about the degree of activation or inhibition of the promoter. The reporter genes that are most commonly used are CAT (chloramphenicol acetyltransferase), LUC (Luciferase), GAL (β-galactosidase) *etc.*

Despite revealing important information regarding the compound at the transcriptional level, this assay also has a disadvantage. This assay requires a long incubation period to allow transcription and translation, which is very tedious.

Second Messenger Assay

Detects the expression of a messenger molecule within a pathway. It is mostly used to target the GPCR's. It works on the principle that if the desired target activates the intracellular calcium storage, its activity can be directly assayed using calcium-sensitive dyes such as Fluo3 and Fluo4. Its advantage over the reporter gene assay is that it has a fast response time (within a fraction of seconds).

Two Hybrid Screening

In this assay, there is a bait protein and a prey protein. Bait protein is allowed to couple with the DNA binding domain while the prey protein attaches to the transcription activation domain. A reporter gene is allowed to get inserted after the promoter region. In this assay, if the prey protein binds to the bait, the transcription activation domain is brought near the reporter gene, which gets activated and is detected [17].

Protein Fragment Complementation Assay

PCA splits the detection protein, in this case, luciferase, GFP, and GAL, into two parts that are fused to the protein-protein interaction partners of interest; if the partners bind, the detection protein is re-formed, and a signal is detected.

Ultra High Throughput Screening (uHTS)-

This is the latest method which screens more than 100,000 compounds at a lower cost in comparison to the traditional assays and is also not much time-consuming. Many compounds can be screened against a single target in almost no time.

High Content Screening (HCS)

It is the most popular HTS used nowadays and is really informative. The instrument used for HCS is highly automated and can read 4 different fluorescence. The HCS instrument automatically collects images from the multi-well plate in which the cells are grown. These images are later analysed for desired measures or the required measures.

Quantitative High Throughput Screening (qHTS)

It is a modified HTS technique that identifies compounds with a wide range of activities. It is a precise method, with accurate profiling of every compound present in the library. It even provides a platform for chemical genomics, thereby accelerating the identification of leads for drug discovery. It generates a database that can be easily compared to identify compounds with a narrow and wide range of spectra of bioactivity, even the ones that are not modulated in the current libraries. The usage of qHTS made the screening of large chemical libraries technically demanding and easier [18].

HTS METHODS FOR SCREENING OF KNOWN DRUGS AGAINST COVID-19

The outbreak of the novel coronavirus in the year 2019 led to a pandemic situation in 2020 in the entire globe. People were losing lives all across the globe. No place was spared by this deadly coronavirus. The high impact of COVID-19 and the lack of commercially available drugs and vaccines against this deadly disease led to the idea of repurposing the already existing FDA-approved drugs to treat the disease [19].

The process of a new drug to be approved is expensive and can take more than 10 years, which is really a long time. So, it is necessary to discover new strategies to reduce drug discovery time. The alternative for drug discovery is drug repurposing. Drug repurposing allows new therapeutic use of the already available drugs in the market [20]. Available drugs are being tested for their antiviral and immunotherapeutic activity against SARS-CoV-2. Repurposing an already existing drug for alternative use is cost-effective and is also a faster process as it has already been clinically tested, and its pharmacokinetics have already been established. There is an urgent need to find assays in order to screen potential compounds present in the libraries that could target SARS-CoV-2. Fig. (**7**) shows diagrammatically how repurposed drugs undergo approval for clinical use.

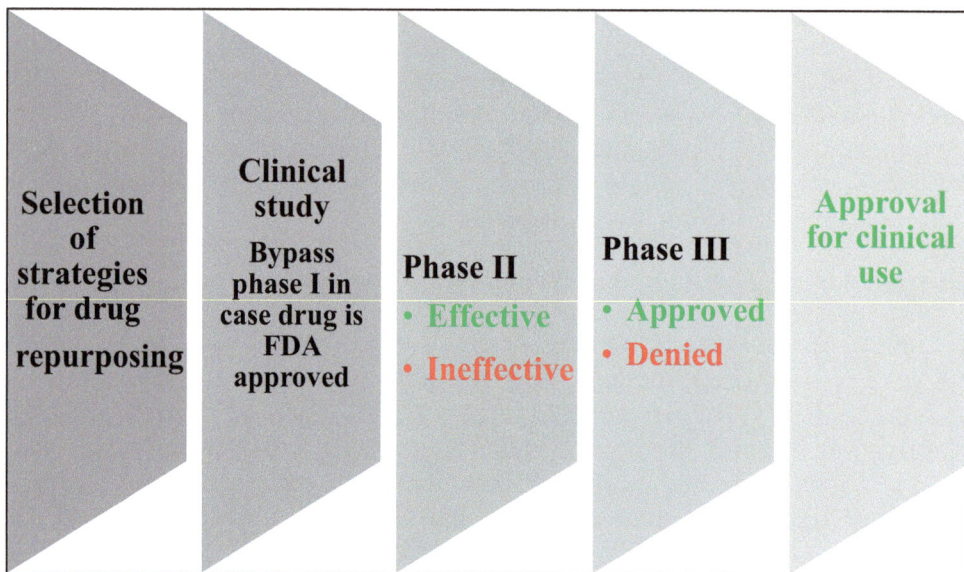

Fig. (7). The selection procedure of already approved drugs for alternative use.

Some existing drugs have been repurposed for the treatment of the COVID-19 patients; some have antiviral activity, some hinders/stalls the viral replication, while some target the enzymes required for viral transmission. They have been found to be effective against COVID-19. The drugs used against COVID-19 are Remdesivir, Hydrocloroquine, Lopinami and Ritonavir. The assays performed for the alternative usage of the drugs are mentioned hereby (Table **1**).

Plaque Reduction Neutralization Test (PRNT)

The PRNT assay is used in the diagnosis of the neutralizing antibody, which is the measure of the immunity of an individual after the COVID-19 infection. It has a long reading time and low throughput screening, making it impossible to diagnose at a large scale. It has a low sensitivity diagnosis. It takes almost 3 days for the diagnosis, which is really time taking [21].

Nanoluciferase SARS-CoV-2 Assay

This assay has been developed to measure the neutralizing antibody as it is the only way to determine the protective immunity of an individual who is previously infected with COVID-19. It has been described as the gold standard method of serological diagnosis. It measures the neutralizing Ab, which is required to block viral replication. It is a reliable antiviral screening. It has a higher sensitivity in comparison to the PRNT assay. It even reduces the diagnosis time from 3days to 5 hours. It even has an increased testing capacity, making it an important assay for the diagnosis at a large scale. Drugs such as Remdesivir and Chloroquine have been screened and validated using this particular assay [21].

Remdesivir is a nucleotide analogue that is known to block viral replication as it interferes with the RNA-dependent RNA polymerase enzyme and stalls the viral replication, and therefore, the viral infection is stalled. Remdesivir is a prodrug that gets metabolized in the host body, its ultimate metabolism leads to a nucleotide analogue which interferes with viral replication. Rupintrivir and Chloroquine are *in vitro* inhibitors of SARS-CoV-2, a potent treatment of SARS-CoV-2.

Pseudotyped Particle Entry Assay

In this assay, a pseudotyped particle (PP) is created using the spike protein of SARS-CoV-2 and a luciferase reporter RNA, surrounded by a bilayer of murine leukemia virus (MLV) gag polymerase. This PP was introduced in the cell. Upon successful entry of the luciferase reporter gene, a luminescence signal is detected. This assay was used to screen many compounds, and the compounds which did not show a luminescence signal were selected as the inhibitor of the SARS-CoV-2

[22]. This pseudotyped particle entry assay is robust for the HTS and can be used for lead discovery. It can be used to screen multiple targets involved in viral entry. It is used to examine the neutralizing Ab and other biologics that block the spike protein of SARS-CoV-2 [23].

In-cell ELISA (icELISA)

It is a cheap, fast, reliable and automated assay for the diagnosis of the neutralizing AB (icNT). The entire assay can be processed in less than 2 days. It provides increased quality of data. It does not require any microscopic detection [24].

TMPRSS2 Biochemical Assay

This assay was used to identify the inhibitors of the TMPRSS2 (Transmembrane Protease Serine 2). TMPRSS2 is known to mediate the fusion of spike protein of SARS-CoV-2. The inhibition of the TMPRSS2 would inhibit the viral fusion, thereby viral entry and thus the infection. Out of the few compounds that were screened, Nafamostat is the most potent drug that inhibits the transmembrane protease serine 2. But the drug is still under clinical trials [25].

3CL^{pro} Activity Assay

Sars-CoV-2 genome is known to encode the 3C-like protease and is responsible for destructing the host proteins, and it is also responsible for the viral polyprotein. This assay targets the activity of 3CL^{pro,} which can also be used as a marker of SARS-CoV-2 replication [26]. A cleavage site is there, which is maintained by the luciferase in an inactive form. In this assay, the cleavage site is processed by the 3CL^{pro} and cleaves into two fragments. Breaking of fragments leads to the bioluminescent activity, which is recorded [27].

This assay can be used to screen large chemical libraries. Vidofludimus, an inhibitor of Dihydroorotate dehydrogenase (DHODH), is reported to inhibit SARS-CoV-2 replication.

Cell-based Assay-Fluorescence Microscopy

Setanaxib has been reported to have antiviral effects. This was confirmed using fluorescence microscopy. This has been known to strongly inhibit the production of viral particles.

For this assay, the SARS-CoV-2 is expressed with mNeon Green. The cells were seeded in a 96-well plate and infected with SARS-CoV-2 expressed mNeon Green and were incubated. Later, the chemical library compounds were added to the plate at different concentrations, followed by incubation. The plate was checked using fluorescence microscopy. The compounds which inhibited the viral entry into the cells did not show fluorescence, while the compounds which could not inhibit the viral entry showed fluorescence. Setanaxib is one the compound which inhibits viral entry into the cell [27].

Other Drugs

Some drugs were earlier used in treating some other diseases, but after undergoing clinical trial, they are directly used for the treatment of COVID-19 disease, as they have anti-viral effects or inhibit the replication of virus. Some of the below-mentioned drugs were directly tested on the hospitalized patients, and, when found effective, came into regular use.

1. **Nafamostat Mesylate** used in combination with **favipiravir** is used to treat critically ill COVID-19 patients. Nafamostat mesylate is a serine protease inhibitor, while favipiravir is the anti-influenza H1N1 virus drug. This drug combination blocks viral entry as well as viral replication [28].

2. **Flavipiravir**- a nucleoside analogue, is found to inhibit RNA-dependent RNA polymerase. Earlier it was used as anti-influenza drug in Japan. It received an emergency approval for the treatment of SARS-CoV-2 disease.

3. **Tocilizumab**-in case of COVID-19, the IL-6 gets elevated, which clearly suggests immune dysfunction. This drug is a monoclonal antibody against IL-6 receptor. It has undergone clinical trials and has been found to be effective against SARS-CoV-2 infection [29].

Table 1. Showing the drugs for COVID-19 and the HTS methods used.

Serial no	Compound	HTS Method Used	Mode of Action/Target Site
1	Remdesivir	Nanoluciferase SARS-CoV-2 assay	Stalls viral replication
2	Setanaxib	Cell based-fluorescence microscopy	Inhibits viral entry
3	Vidofludimus	3CL^{pro} activity assay	Inhibits viral replication
4	Nafamostat	TMPRSS2 biochemical assay	Inhibits TMPRSS2
5	Chloroquine	Nanoluciferase SARS-CoV-2 assay	Inhibits viral replication

Advantages of HTS

The High Throughput Screening has been a supportive and cooperative technique in this time of the pandemic. The technique has been used for a long time and continuously develops and modifies according to the need and requirement. Ever since its development, those technique has been really useful in the process of drug development. Within less time, it allows us to get a lead molecule for the development of the drug against the disease, which, when done manually, could take a really long time and could be tiresome as well. Earlier HTS techniques could take a long time and also require a lot of patience and experience.

HTS technology has continuously developed itself with time, and now the processing time has reduced and contributed to the improvement of the existing assays. With time, the detection methods have also improved. Now virtual screening is used in the process of HTS. In HTS, the data sequence can be analysed by multiple end-users and can also be reanalysed as the database is expanded [30]. More recent advancement in this technique is the ultra HTS, which takes very less time in comparison to the traditional HTS technology. The advantage of HTS is that low-volume dispensing could be done easily. This technique uses high-sensitivity detectors with robotic plate handling, which could be less time-consuming.

Challenges in HTS Technology

Since 1980's, HTS has faced a lot of challenges and these challenges compelled me to come out with something new and effective every time. During 1980's, 10,000 compounds were screened per year, which was time taking and not at all cost-effective. With the development of technology, in the early 1990's, 10,000 compounds were screened per month per target, which was much better than the HTS technologies used earlier. During the mid 1990's, due to advancements in HTS technology, a lot of compounds were screened per week, taking much less time and was also cost-effective. Traditional drug discovery methods would take years for the production of a single drug [5].

The major challenge faced by the HTS technology was time and cost, which was later overcome by the latest technologies. The radiometric assays were replaced by fluorescent ones for easy detection. The technologies that developed over time were easy to handle, had improved technologies and were even user-friendly. Earlier the HTS was done manually, which took longer than usual time, but with the advancement in HTS technology, the time taking reduced, and machines became automated and user-friendly software that could be easily handled. In the 1980's, the sensitivity of HTS was not good, but with time, we now have better sensitivity. The biological assays were not too good for detection, but with time, the assays have improved much. We now have enhanced compound libraries. Searching for an effective lead discovery was a real challenge in the early days, but now the effectiveness has increased with improved assays and detection methods. Development of new tools is one of the major challenges as the cost of instrumentation is too high. Another important challenge in HTS is analysing the data. It needs a lot of patience, professionalism and dedication for the keen analysis of the data. There may be chances of a low hit rate due to incompatible libraries selected [31].

Future Perspective

Pharmaceutical companies are nowadays largely dependent on HTS technology. Improvement in software and biological assays is expected to develop soon. Successful primary screening is expected in the future, which costs less. In the future, miniaturization of liquid handlings, such as micro-fluids, is expected. The future perspective of HTS is improved biological assays with better automation tools and improved software.

Unmet Needs in Case of Screening

The major requirement that needs to be developed in the near future is biological assays. The second things that come into consideration are the data management tools and the automation and productivity of the technology. We need more compound libraries which shall be helpful in finding the "hit" compound. The other thing that is the need of an hour is better detection methods. It also includes the improvement in biological assays. The other need of the hour includes validation of the target. In the future, the miniaturization is expected to reduce [32]. In the future, along with miniaturization, we also expect to use low volume, higher sensitivity and other advanced techniques, making this technique more friendly and less time-consuming.

The HTS technology has been using immortalized cells for the process of drug discovery, but there are some technical difficulties in using stem cells (embryonic or adult stem cells). In the future, HTS should develop some feasible technologies that could use these stem cells for the purpose of target validation without any technical difficulties [33].

Various Methods used for Target Identification

The HTS screens hundreds to thousands of compounds to get a target compound with desired characteristics which are known as "hits". The major goal of HTS is to get a target compound. For this, various methods are there which allow target identification. Appropriate analytical methods have been adopted for "hit" selection.

The basic tools for the identification of the target area are as below Fig. (**8**).

• Genomics

• Proteomics

• Bioinformatics

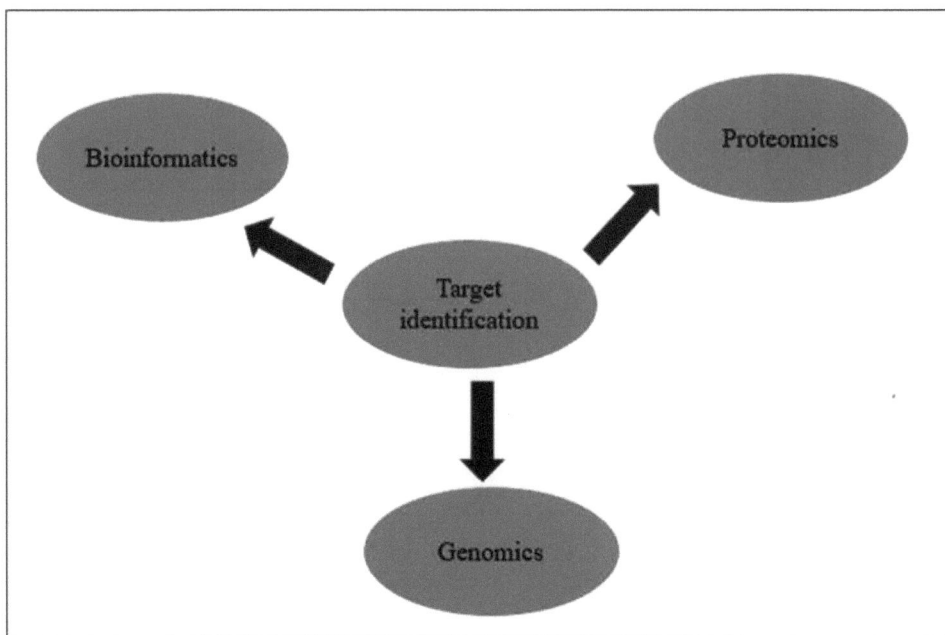

Fig. (8). Shows the tools of target identification.

Genomics is the field of science that deals with an organism's genome, focusing on its structure and function. It is concerned with the sequencing and analysis of organisms. Majorly genomics has two subgroups- structural genomics and functional genomics. Structural genomics provides information about the structure of the protein in the desired target, while structural genomics deals with the transcriptional and translational regulations of the gene.

Proteomics is the field that deals with the protein present in the cells or tissues of an organism. The HTS method exploits proteomics to study the interaction of the proteins as well the activity of the protein, whether it is getting activated or inhibited. The third tool is one the most important part of target identification. It is used to analyze the data and study the sequence of the target and explain the observed mutation that occurs in nature.

CONCLUSION

This book chapter includes information regarding the high throughput screening and the HTS methods that have been used in identifying the drugs for the treatment of the COVID-19 disease. The HTS method is a really useful and robust method for screening hundreds to thousands of compounds against a single target. The HTS allows us to identify a single compound with desired characteristics against the target. The identified compound is then allowed to undergo validation, where they are assayed for the required purpose.

Since the 1980s, a lot of progress has been seen in the methods of HTS and the assays used for optimization. With time and need, HTS methods have become automated, less costly, and consume less time. But still, a lot is needed to be done in this field. Some assays take a longer time for detection and are really costly, so these assays should be targeted to make them cost-effective and try to reduce the detection time. With time, technology is advancing, and new automated devices are being developed as well; the only limitation is the cost and miniaturization of these techniques.

The compound libraries need to be sorted into different groups, such as structure, target, function, genome sequence *etc.* this will make it easier for the target identification, which is the initial and the most important step of drug delivery, in order to make virtual screening more important. HTS includes machine learning, computational pattern recognition as well as statistical modelling [34]. In the future, we should expect more enhancement in the development of the HTS methods, which can screen more than thousands of compounds against a single target within no time.

LIST OF ABBREVIATIONS

SARS-CoV-2	Severe Acute Respiratory Syndrome Coronavirus-2
Covid 19	Coronavirus 19
HTS	High Throughput Screening
uHTS	Ultra High Throughput Screening
NMR	Nuclear Magnetic Resonance
DSF	Differential Scanning Fluorimetry
SPA	Scintillating Proximity Assay
FA/FP	Fluorescence Anisotropy/Fluorescence Polarization
FRET	Fluorescence Resonance Energy Transfer
FCS	Fluorescence Correlation Spectroscopy

TR-FRET	Time Resolve-FRET
Ln+3	Lanthanide complex
FBDD	Fragment Based Drug Design
SPR	Surface Plasmin Resonance
CAT	Chloramphenicol acetyl transferase
LUC	Luciferase
GAL	B-galactosidase
GPCRs	G-protein coupled receptors
PCA	Protein fragment complementation assay
HCS	High content screening
PRNT	Plaque Reduction Neutralization Test
PP	Pseudotyped particle
MLV	Murine Leukemia Virus
icELISA	In cell Enzyme Linked Immuno Sorbant Assay
TMPRSS2	Transmembrane Protease Serine 2
DHODH	Dihydroorodate Dehydrogenase
FDA	Food and development authority
NPC	NCATS Pharmaceutical collection
MIPE	Mechanism interrogation plate
NPACT	NCATS pharmacologically active chemical toolbox
NCATS	National Center for Advancing Translational Sciences
qHTS	Quantitative High Throughput Screening

CONSENT FOR PUBLICATION

Not applicable.

CONFLICT OF INTEREST

The author declares no conflict of interest, financial or otherwise.

ACKNOWLEDGEMENTS

We would like to thank our institutions Biological Research Centre, University of Szeged, Szeged, Hungary and SRM University for providing a supportive environment to carry out this work.

REFERENCES

[1]   Hughes JP, Rees S, Kalindjian SB, Philpott KL. Principles of early drug discovery. Br J Pharmacol

2011; 162(6): 1239-49.
[http://dx.doi.org/10.1111/j.1476-5381.2010.01127.x] [PMID: 21091654]

[2]   Lloyd MD. High-throughput screening for the discovery of enzyme inhibitors. J Med Chem 2020; 63(19): 10742-72.
[http://dx.doi.org/10.1021/acs.jmedchem.0c00523] [PMID: 32432874]

[3]   Carnero A. High throughput screening in drug discovery. Clin Transl Oncol 2006; 8(7): 482-90.
[http://dx.doi.org/10.1007/s12094-006-0048-2] [PMID: 16870538]

[4]   Kontoyianni M. Docking and virtual screening in drug discovery InProteomics for drug discovery 2017; 255-66.

[5]   Dick AS, Basu K. from the SAGE Social Science Collections. All Rights Hisp J Behav Sci 1987; 9(2): 183-205.

[6]   Entzeroth M, Flotow H, Condron P. Overview of high-throughput screening. Curr Protocols Pharmacol 2009; Chapter 9(1): 4.
[PMID: 22294406]

[7]   Pereira DA, Williams JA. Origin and evolution of high throughput screening. Br J Pharmacol 2007; 152(1): 53-61.
[http://dx.doi.org/10.1038/sj.bjp.0707373] [PMID: 17603542]

[8]   Gong Z, Hu G, Li Q, *et al.* Compound libraries: recent advances and their applications in drug discovery. Curr Drug Discov Technol 2017; 14(4): 216-28.
[http://dx.doi.org/10.2174/1570163814666170425155154] [PMID: 28443514]

[9]   Owicki JC. Fluorescence polarization and anisotropy in high throughput screening: perspectives and primer. SLAS Discov 2000; 5(5): 297-306.
[http://dx.doi.org/10.1177/108705710000500501] [PMID: 11080688]

[10]   Hall MD, Yasgar A, Peryea T, *et al.* Fluorescence polarization assays in high-throughput screening and drug discovery: a review. Methods Appl Fluoresc 2016; 4(2): 022001.
[http://dx.doi.org/10.1088/2050-6120/4/2/022001] [PMID: 28809163]

[11]   Vedel L, Bräuner-Osborne H, Mathiesen JM. A cAMP biosensor-based high-throughput screening assay for identification of Gs-coupled GPCR ligands and phosphodiesterase inhibitors. SLAS Discov 2015; 20(7): 849-57.
[http://dx.doi.org/10.1177/1087057115580019] [PMID: 25851033]

[12]   Blay V, Tolani B, Ho SP, Arkin MR. High-Throughput Screening: today's biochemical and cell-based approaches. Drug Discov Today 2020; 25(10): 1807-21.
[http://dx.doi.org/10.1016/j.drudis.2020.07.024] [PMID: 32801051]

[13]   Wachsmuth M, Conrad C, Bulkescher J, *et al.* High-throughput fluorescence correlation spectroscopy enables analysis of proteome dynamics in living cells. Nat Biotechnol 2015; 33(4): 384-9.
[http://dx.doi.org/10.1038/nbt.3146] [PMID: 25774713]

[14]   Fu X, Song Y, Masud A, Nuti K, DeRouchey JE, Richards CI. High-throughput fluorescence correlation spectroscopy enables analysis of surface components of cell-derived vesicles. Anal Bioanal Chem 2020; 412(11): 2589-97.
[http://dx.doi.org/10.1007/s00216-020-02485-z] [PMID: 32146499]

[15]   Wang T, Wu MB, Chen ZJ, Chen H, Lin JP, Yang LR. Fragment-based drug discovery and molecular docking in drug design. Curr Pharm Biotechnol 2015; 16(1): 11-25.
[http://dx.doi.org/10.2174/1389201015666141122204532] [PMID: 25420726]

[16]   Joseph-McCarthy D, Campbell AJ, Kern G, Moustakas D. Fragment-based lead discovery and design. J Chem Inf Model 2014; 54(3): 693-704.
[http://dx.doi.org/10.1021/ci400731w] [PMID: 24490951]

[17]   Suter B, Wanker EE. The investigation of binary PPIs with the classical yeast two-hybrid (Y2H)

approach, Y2H variants, and other *in vivo* methods for PPI mapping. Methods Mol Biol 2012; 812: v-vi.
[http://dx.doi.org/10.1007/978-1-61779-455-1] [PMID: 22319789]

[18]   Inglese J, Auld DS, Jadhav A, *et al.* Quantitative high-throughput screening: A titration-based approach that efficiently identifies biological activities in large chemical libraries. Proc Natl Acad Sci USA 2006; 103(31): 11473-8.
[http://dx.doi.org/10.1073/pnas.0604348103] [PMID: 16864780]

[19]   Park JG, Oladunni FS, Chiem K, *et al.* Rapid *in vitro* assays for screening neutralizing antibodies and antivirals against SARS-CoV-2. J Virol Methods 2021; 287: 113995.
[http://dx.doi.org/10.1016/j.jviromet.2020.113995] [PMID: 33068703]

[20]   Parvathaneni V, Kulkarni NS, Muth A, Gupta V. Drug repurposing: a promising tool to accelerate the drug discovery process. Drug Discov Today 2019; 24(10): 2076-85.
[http://dx.doi.org/10.1016/j.drudis.2019.06.014] [PMID: 31238113]

[21]   Xie X, Muruato AE, Zhang X, *et al.* A nanoluciferase SARS-CoV-2 for rapid neutralization testing and screening of anti-infective drugs for COVID-19. Nat Commun 2020; 11(1): 5214.
[http://dx.doi.org/10.1038/s41467-020-19055-7] [PMID: 33060595]

[22]   Xu M, Pradhan M, Gorshkov K, *et al.* A high throughput screening assay for inhibitors of SARS-Co--2 pseudotyped particle entry. SLAS Discov 2022; 27(2): 86-94.
[http://dx.doi.org/10.1016/j.slasd.2021.12.005] [PMID: 35086793]

[23]   Hu J, Gao Q, He C, Huang A, Tang N, Wang K. Development of cell-based pseudovirus entry assay to identify potential viral entry inhibitors and neutralizing antibodies against SARS-CoV-2. Genes Dis 2020; 7(4): 551-7.
[http://dx.doi.org/10.1016/j.gendis.2020.07.006] [PMID: 32837985]

[24]   Schöler L, Le-Trilling VTK, Eilbrecht M, *et al.* A Novel in-cell ELISA assay allows rapid and automated quantification of SARS-CoV-2 to analyze neutralizing antibodies and antiviral compounds. Front Immunol 2020; 11: 573526.
[http://dx.doi.org/10.3389/fimmu.2020.573526] [PMID: 33162987]

[25]   Shrimp JH, Kales SC, Sanderson PE, Simeonov A, Shen M, Hall MD. An enzymatic TMPRSS2 assay for assessment of clinical candidates and discovery of inhibitors as potential treatment of COVID-19. ACS Pharmacol Transl Sci 2020; 3(5): 997-1007.
[http://dx.doi.org/10.1021/acsptsci.0c00106] [PMID: 33062952]

[26]   Ma C, Sacco MD, Xia Z, *et al.* Discovery of SARS-CoV-2 Papain-like Protease Inhibitors through a Combination of High-Throughput Screening and a FlipGFP-Based Reporter Assay. ACS Cent Sci 2021; 7(7): 1245-60.
[http://dx.doi.org/10.1021/acscentsci.1c00519] [PMID: 34341772]

[27]   Mathieu C, Touret F, Jacquemin C, *et al.* A Bioluminescent 3CL^{Pro} Activity Assay to Monitor SARS-CoV-2 Replication and Identify Inhibitors. Viruses 2021; 13(9): 1814.
[http://dx.doi.org/10.3390/v13091814] [PMID: 34578395]

[28]   Ikeda M, Hayase N, Moriya K, Morimura N. Nafamostat mesylate treatment in combination with favipiravir for patients critically ill with Covid-19: a case series. Crit Care 2020; 24(1): 1-4.
[PMID: 31898531]

[29]   Rosas IO, Bräu N, Waters M, *et al.* Tocilizumab in hospitalized patients with severe Covid-19 pneumonia. N Engl J Med 2021; 384(16): 1503-16.
[http://dx.doi.org/10.1056/NEJMoa2028700] [PMID: 33631066]

[30]   Maree HJ, Fox A, Al Rwahnih M, Boonham N, Candresse T. Application of HTS for routine plant virus diagnostics: state of the art and challenges. Front Plant Sci 2018; 9: 1082.
[http://dx.doi.org/10.3389/fpls.2018.01082] [PMID: 30210506]

[31]   Dunn DA, Feygin I. Challenges and solutions to ultra-high-throughput screening assay

miniaturization: submicroliter fluid handling. Drug Discov Today 2000; 5(12) (Suppl. 1): 84-91.
[http://dx.doi.org/10.1016/S1359-6446(00)00064-7] [PMID: 11564571]

[32]   Mayr LM, Fuerst P. The future of high-throughput screening. SLAS Discov 2008; 13(6): 443-8.
[http://dx.doi.org/10.1177/1087057108319644] [PMID: 18660458]

[33]   Eglen R, Reisine T. Primary cells and stem cells in drug discovery: emerging tools for high-throughput
screening. Assay Drug Dev Technol 2011; 9(2): 108-24.
[http://dx.doi.org/10.1089/adt.2010.0305] [PMID: 21186936]

[34]   Kundu B. High throughput technologies in drug discovery. Comb Chem High Throughput Screen
2011; 14(10): 829.
[http://dx.doi.org/10.2174/138620711797537094] [PMID: 21843140]

[35]   https://www.ddw-online.com/needs-and-challenges-in-high-throughput-screening-554-200712/

CHAPTER 7

Drug Repurposing for COVID-19 using Computational Methods

Om Prakash[1] and **Feroz Khan**[1,*]

[1] *Technology Dissemination and Computational Biology Division, CSIR-Central Institute of Medicinal & Aromatic Plants, P.O.-CIMAP, Kukrail Picnic Spot Road, Lucknow-226015 (Uttar Pradesh), India*

Abstract: In this chapter, we use computational methods to illustrate drug repurposing with the example of COVID-19. Here, the current status of drug discovery has been described with various aspects of drug repurposing interactions, use of algorithms in drug repurposing, re-evaluation of existing drugs, challenges in drug repurposing, and biological and computational interpretation of personalised and AI-guided repurposing. In addition, we present blueprints for pacing up the drug repurposing process using artificial intelligence. This chapter is devoted to the use of computational intelligence for drug repurposing against various diseases, including COVID-19.

Keywords: Artificial intelligence, Computational methods, COVID-19, Drug, Repurposing.

INTRODUCTION

Multiple drugs have been developed for various diseases [1]. The majority of them were discovered by serendipity. This process developed a huge collection of approved drugs, which provides an opportunity to rethink the purposes of drugs in various human physiological statuses. In today's scenario, re-thinking about the purpose of drugs is termed "Drug repurposing" [2]. It is a thematic terminology, representing a way of working for identification of those suggestive clues, which can provide a strong ground for rethinking the purpose of exiting or pipelined drugs. The back force for such repurposing comes due to the bonus benefit of getting rid of a major part of clinical trials; which may become very supportive for saving time & money, as well as approaching new prescriptions to the patients in a very cost-effective manner [2]. The theme of repurposing is not new; for decades, researchers have already been devoted to reviewing the aspects of

---

* **Corresponding author Feroz Khan:** Technology Dissemination and Computational Biology Division, CSIR-Central Institute of Medicinal & Aromatic Plants, P.O.-CIMAP, Kukrail Picnic Spot Road, Lucknow-226015 (Uttar Pradesh), India; E-mail: f.khan@cimap.res.in

existing drugs for various utilities. In this way, research outputs from previous studies became the ground for cultivating the idea for the identification of additional usage of previous studies [3].

Multiple reports are available, which show the success story as well as existing challenges regarding drug repurposing. Success represents the power of drug repurposing for fast drug identification for newly developing diseases, also useful for searching for solutions in pandemic situations. But, background information about molecular interactions with newly developing drugs is always challenging. Because molecular interactions follow relative behavior, a complete set of a system of molecular components is required to understand the behavior of each drug molecule. For such types of studies, the genomic ground is required to agitate the combinations of system properties to extract significant therapeutic interpretations. On the coarse side of such observations, attempts have been implemented with various interactomes to understand and interpret computational drug development. To handle the complexity of data analysis, algorithms from artificial intelligence were used for drug repurposing. These efforts of understanding the interactions are used for finding the hidden aspects, as well as unravelling the possible links among various drugs, targets, and human diseases. Such clues become very important for resolving possible drug repurposing. This seems possible because of the sharable functional behavior of protein-protein interactions, which shows that drug targeting for one disease may resolve another too [4].

About Data Size & its Handling with Computational Methods: Long-term experimental practices, dumped huge electronic data. Using such large data for rethinking any drug based on stored experimental data, the existence of false negatives is quite feasible. Therefore, handling big data requires high-end applications of information technology. In the mid-19th century, researchers had forecasted computational methods as an approval ground for human interpretations. These enhancements are only possible with artificial intelligence. When we consider forecasting for repurposing, AI dependencies also come into existence. Computation for such machine intelligence requires a high computation capacity of processors as well as high storage capacity. Concrete establishment in artificial intelligence, based on the novel wealth of data, is only feasible with high processing and storage capacity. Now it is well known that artificial intelligence is being implemented in diverse areas of research as well as technological developments in the area of data mining. Artificial intelligence is also revolutionizing the area of drug discovery by exposing patterns from biological data. The existing R&D units use artificial intelligence for computational drug discovery and development. These technologies define diseases and their therapeutic aspects with minimum error [5].

This chapter introduces methods implemented for drug repurposing in general. Specific explanations of drug-repurposing were also provided with examples of COVID-19. Here, we discuss the current status in drug discovery, approaches already implemented for drug repurposing, computational methods used in drug repurposing, information about possible existing drugs used during pandemic conditions, challenges faced during drug repurposing, Biological and non-biological criteria for handling personalized and Artificial Intelligence-guided repurposing. We also attempted to present a clear picture of the possible utilization of AI for speeding up drug repurposing. This chapter provides a strong rationale for drug repurposing against various human diseases, including COVID-19.

CURRENT STATUS OF DRUG-REPURPOSING

Drug repurposing is one of the enhancing ways of identifying new therapeutic molecules. Diversified utilization of various methods has been implemented for the discovery of drugs in the most efficient way. Methods used involve structure-based processes for the identification of drugs, *i.e.*, involving structures of ligands and proteins. Now the question arises of how to relate the combinations of structures for drug-repurposing. The point of attention is that the purpose of drugs can be represented by either structure of drug, or structure of protein, or both. The reason behind this is that here, repurposing is dependent on the known structures (*i.e.*, drugs and proteins) and their biological functionality. That means any type of link between drug and protein will present their existing relationships as in any standard network. Therefore, if our analysis process somehow re-establishes links between the drugs and proteins, then it will represent the repurposing of drugs. Now, the question arises, how many ways can present the interactions of drugs & proteins. Ultimately by implementing the structure-functionality linking, we have to perform a screening process for drug repurposing. Till now, docking followed by molecular dynamics-based virtual screening was the method for structure-function-based screening. Now, big-data-based structure-functionality linking has become the evolving method for establishing an efficient way for screening molecules for possible functionalities. Here, we will discuss the linking-based content for drug-repurposing-based methods one by one [6].

Repurposing Through a Drug-drug Interaction Network

One way to observe drug repurposing may be the observation of drug-drug interactions. This process is based on pharmacological functions (PhFs). PhFs can be used as selective behavior of drugs for specific purposes because drugs with similar PhFs will be compactly clustered at one centroid, while non-clustered drugs may be picked for suitable re-purposing. These PhFs can be defined based on drug interaction information collected from DrugBank. As if we cluster PhFs along with the drug information, the un-clustered PhFs will represent indications towards possible potential repositioning. In a study [7], a drug-drug interaction network has been developed based on PhFs. Network nodes were clustered based on modularity and force-directed layout. Clustered drugs showed 09 specific drug properties. The main attention was made to the topology placed in the bordering zones of the clusters. About 15% of drugs were found at the cluster border, showing hints of repurposing.

Other studies investigating the potential of using non-antibiotic drugs as antibiotic adjuvants have exposed the art of repurposing non-antibiotic drugs as potential adjuvants with discussions on classification and mechanism of action. This was reported as a novel screening platform. Similarly, the use of big data analysis from clinical sources is also explored for discovering new and unanticipated hypotheses based on drug-drug interactions that lead to drug repositioning [8]. The combination of these results was reported to define curated drug-miRNA associations using a comprehensive drug-drug interaction network. Other studies re-used the drug-drug interaction network to determine new associations. The data used involved properties of drug molecules, drug-target binding, drug-drug interactions, drug-induced gene expression, and data on drug-induced therapeutic effects and side effects. This method only focuses on diagnosing and classifying drug-drug interactions. To develop a new drug efficiently, one needs a machine that integrates viral kinetics with pharmacokinetics. There are, however, drug-drug interactions that suggest some of the drugs used to treat COVID-19 may affect the drug metabolism of anticancer therapies, which could lead to adverse drug reactions [9]. To reduce the number of potential adverse events, drug-drug interactions, and cost while maintaining a sustained antiviral effect, consideration was given to repositioning antiretroviral therapy into combination therapies. In the case of treatment of patients with seizures along with COVID-19, potential drug-drug interactions-based therapies were used with anti-seizure medications as well as mechanisms of COVID-19 action [10].

Repurposing through a Drug-target Interaction Network

Another way to observe possibilities for drug repurposing, may be an observation of drug-target interactions. Drug-target networks are the basis of pharmaceutical innovations. All possible combinations of drugs vs. targets are used for this purpose. The main challenge in this way is the establishment of a method for defining drug-target combinations [11].

Experimental methods used to determine drug-target interactions are often time-consuming, tedious, expensive, and sometimes not reproducible, which is why finding molecular interactions is an essential step in the early phases repurposing. To facilitate the development of the drug repositioning field, new bioinformatics approaches to the prediction of drug-target interactions, continuous updates of the databases, and the development of novel validation techniques are necessary. To suggest new drug candidates or reposition old drugs, the prediction of drug-target interactions (DTIs) is of enormous importance to modern drug discovery [12]. To increase clinical efficiency and productivity during drug discovery and development, network-aided *in silico* approaches are widely used for predicting drug-target interactions and evaluating drug safety. Researchers were able to derive various computational methods to determine unknown drug-target interactions due to the availability of heterogeneous biological data. Several types of data were used, including the properties of chemical structures, therapeutic effects and side effects, binding properties of drugs to target cells, drug-drug interactions, and bioactivity data for molecules across multiple biological targets and drug-induced gene expressions, for defining drug-target interaction. Molecular docking and machine learning-based methods are also reported in a study for predicting drug-target interactions.

Repurposing Through Drug Pairwise Similarity

Another method, synonymous with Drug-Target combination, is observing pairwise similarity based on profile defined based on the structure of drug & target feature. Pairwise similarity can be calculated by a bipartite graph-based method. It uses molecular as well as chemical features as input; *i.e.*, a weighted sum of structural as well as target interaction profile similarity are used at the same time for calculation of pairwise similarity, followed by prediction of the repurposed drug [13].

Repurposing Through Model Hybridization & Systems Modelling

Model hybridization is another idea for better screening of existing drugs. In a study, a model hybridization technique was used for screening FDA-approved drugs for selective targeting of AKT (Fig. **1**). Similarly, this technique can be used for drug repurposing for antiviral activity, specifically against broad-spectrum variants of COVID-19. Model hybridization technique defines the kinetic merger of two-tier models.

Since, this process utilizes system kinetics, therefore identified molecules need to be further screened through a system model. As in a similar study, identified AKT binding molecules were processed through a mitophagy systems model for anti-apoptotic activity. Similarly, in the case of antiviral activity, screened-out molecules through a hybrid model must be re-evaluated through a host-virus interaction system or similar systems model at the *in-silico* level. The outputs through these processes need to be re-observed through laboratory experiments for the authenticity of the molecules [14].

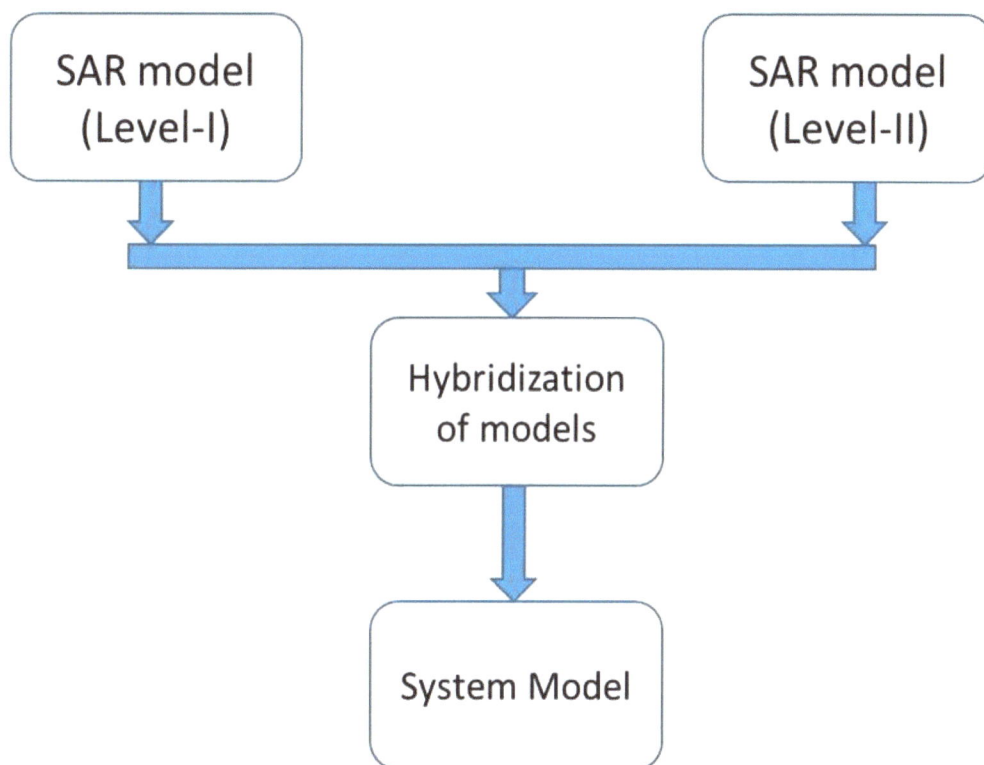

Fig. (1). Drug repurposing through model hybridization and system modeling.

Identification of potential molecules inspired through biological observation of host-virus interaction (*Content accessed through permission of the author with copyright DOI: 10.26434/chemrxiv.12241634.v1*) [15].

It must be the more realistic way to process drug-repurposing if it is performed on the ground of observation through the biological behavior of host-virus interaction. In a study, a biological observation was made by understanding the behavior of Coronaviruses for the interaction of hosts through recognition of 9-O-Ac-sialoglycan. It is a landmark for the entry gate for viruses. Receptor determinant analogs were identified for all glycan-recognizing Coronaviruses, which may mislead viruses for entry into the cell through receptor determinant. Viruses recognise 9-O-Ac-sialoglycan as part of the receptor determinant. In this study, analogs compounds were identified which have similar pharmacophore as

9-O-Ac-sialoglycan. For identification of analogs, virus surface receptor glycoprotein plays a role. Glycoprotein to 9-O-Ac-sialoglycan interaction is the representation of virus-host interaction. This type of interaction has been observed in influenza viruses as well as Coronavirus. This interaction has a molecular conservation domain, which provides host virus interaction selectivity. This conservation become the basis of generation of profile, which can be used as filter to screen compounds from ZINC database (Fig. **2**). The filtered-out molecules were re-observed among the applicability domain defined by existing antiviral drugs as well as natural existing receptor determinants with sialic acid. The identified analogs were:

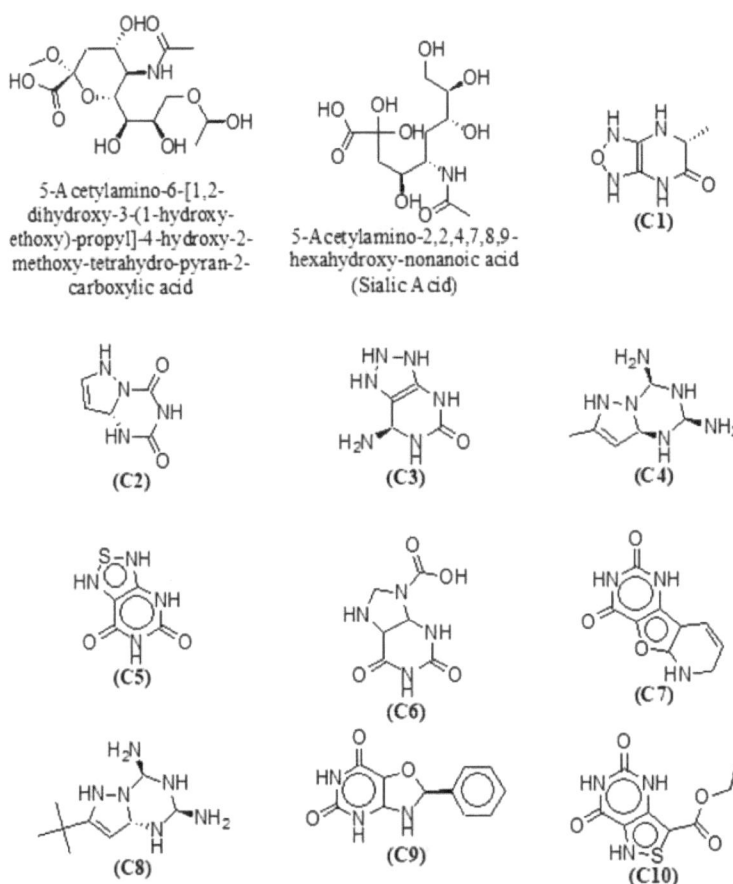

5-Acetylamino-6-[1,2-dihydroxy-3-(1-hydroxy-ethoxy)-propyl]-4-hydroxy-2-methoxy-tetrahydro-pyran-2-carboxylic acid

5-Acetylamino-2,2,4,7,8,9-hexahydroxy-nonanoic acid (Sialic Acid)

(C1)

(C2)   (C3)   (C4)

(C5)   (C6)   (C7)

(C8)   (C9)   (C10)

Fig. (2). Compounds identified through pharmacophore screening of ZINC database.

Here sialic acid was found to be the conserved part from receptor determinant, which become the basis for identification of analogs, which can be recognised by the surface glycoprotein of the receptor with N-acetly-9-O-acetylneuramic acid.

The 9-O-acetyl group of Sialic acid is released by the receptor-destroying enzyme acetylesterase. If analogues are designed to mimic the receptor determinant, then acetylesterase will be unable to act on the analogues, further halting the signalling process for virus entry into the host. It should be noted that the analogues will act as receptor determinants, but they will not protect antiviral performers. Sialic acids are known as receptor determinants for coronaviruses in general.

PDB 6NZK was used to extract the conserved domain of the glycoprotein's groove. The domain contains Asn27, Asp28, Lys29, Asp30, Thr31, Leu80, Lys81, Ser83, Val84, Leu85, Leu86, Trp90, and Phe95 residues. This is divided into two subdomains, P1 and P2. P1 has a hydrophobic pocket with residues at serial numbers 85, 86, and 90, while P2 has residues at serial numbers 80, 90, and 95. 9-O-Ac-sialoglycan, a wild receptor determinant, stacks into the groove. The pharmacophore features were defined using pockets with conserved residues. The pharmacophore had four basic components: a hydrogen bond acceptor, a hydrogen bond donor, hydrophobic areas, and aromatic rings. Three-dimensional orientations of these four features were discovered to be important in defining a pharmacophore equivalent to multiple analogues of receptor determinants. The distance between pharmacophore features was found to range between 1.68 and 3.9 angstrom; hydrophobic locations were found to be the closest, while hydrogen bond acceptors and aromatic rings were found to be the farthest away. Because it filtered out only 10 possible structures from the zinc database, this pharmacophore was discovered to be very selective. C1-10 were assigned to these identified molecules.

The screened-out molecules and antiviral drugs were observed on the basis of LogP and Molecular Weight to visualise the possibilities of the existence of identified molecules within the applicability domain of antiviral drugs. The identified molecules were discovered to be within the same applicability domain defined for antiviral activity. The majority of them fall into the negative LogP range. LogP is a pharmacokinetic property that is used to define drug behaviour during passive diffusion of carrier-mediated uptake. As a result, this property was used to define an applicability domain or a set of molecules for a specific purpose.-The queried molecule can be accessed based on the boundaries of the applicability domain defined by LogP and other pharmacokinetic features. LogP is also well known for assessing the Lipophilicity of chemical compounds, and it is a component of Lipinski's rule of five. Because this property is directly related to the pH-dependent behaviour of compounds within the system's environment, it becomes an important parameter during the drug development process evaluation. The molecular weight of the compound is another factor considered when defining the generalised applicability domain. As a result, LogP and Molecular weight provided a foundation for establishing a framework of evaluation for any small molecule queried for its presence in previously known standard drugs.

Screening Molecules Through Understanding the Kinetics Of Viral-host Interaction (*Content accessed through permission of the author with copyright DOI: 10.26434/chemrxiv.12424376.v1*) [16].

In continuation of the identification of antiviral molecules through biological information, efficacies of the analogs were evaluated through understanding the kinetic behavior of molecular interaction. Hydrophobicity was found as a parameter to quantify the relative efficacy of receptor determinants during host-virus interaction. An analytical description of a moment when a virus's surface protein recognises the surface part (receptor determinants) at the host was used in this study. The successful recognition of a viral infection is the first step in the infection's progression. This newly discovered mechanism is significant because it can be used to create barriers to viral infection. However, the kinetics, as well as the components involved in this brief event, remain unexplored. This study aimed to identify governing parameters and kinetics that can be used to quantify the relative efficiency of various receptor determinant analogues. The study was also used to prioritise receptor determinant analogues for Coronavirus. This protocol model can also be used as an add-on for the theoretical modelling of host cell viral infectivity.

The kinetic model was built around the 'Nelson-Siegel-Svensson' (NSS) model. The kinetics of the interaction between the receptor determinant and the spike groove were defined using this model. Because of similarities discovered between the skeleton of the first derivative of the NSS model and the interaction between receptor determinants and spikes, this model was used to customise. When similarly defined pharmacophore-based small molecules are introduced into the domain of the binding site, their responses vary, which can also be used to define the performance of analogues as receptor determinants. As a result, the key components of the zero rate NSS model were restructured to account for molecular interaction. Finally, the ability of a ligand to chase the viral spike was defined as the ratio of hydrophobicity to impact on the viral spike. The chasing capacity of a ligand-based on hydrophobicity was defined as the absolute value of the difference of LogP and LogD, whereas the impact of hydrophobicity was defined as a function of hydrophobicity and four additional parameters 1, 2, 3, and. Because it is a matter of interference between the virus spike and the human cell, interfering molecules can interact with the spike, allowing the virus to enter the host. To select and customise the kinetics model for the interaction of 'receptor determinant' vs. spike groove, assumptions were made. It was assumed that the pharmacophore requirement would already be met by testing molecules. During testing, the molecule will interact with the target, which is the virus's spike groove; it will then affect the virus with varying degrees of infectivity. Taking these assumptions into account, the Nelson-Siegel-Svensson (NSS) forwarding rate model was modified to define the ligand's ability to chase the virus's spike. Because the receptor, determinant interacts with the conserved pocket for a short period of time, this customised assumption can also be understood as: The duration of the interaction is determined by the degree of hydrophobicity. As a result, it was assumed that chasing efficacy can be defined by the capacity of interaction remaining at the last moment of interaction, which was defined by hydrophobicity. A tenor point is defined by the extent of hydrophobicity defined the last moment of interaction. As a result, in this case, the kinetics rate was defined as the integration of the NSS forward rate up to the tenor point of maximum interaction.

Here Ligand is assumed to be a Receptor determinant analogue.

$$Hydrophobicity\ chasing\ ability\ of\ ligand\ (H)\ =\ abs(logP \sim logD)$$

$$Impact\ of\ H\ on\ Viral\ spike\ (D)\ =\ f(H, \alpha1, \alpha2, \alpha3, \beta)$$

$$D(H)\ =\ \alpha1\ +\ (\alpha2 + \alpha3) * (\beta/H) * (1 - exp(-H/\beta)) - (\alpha3 * exp(-H/\beta))$$

$$\textbf{Ligand's ability to chase Viral Spike}\ =\ H\ /\ D(H)$$

Where values for $\alpha1$, $\alpha2$, $\alpha3$, β will vary according to domain

Finally, the efficacy of ligand can be defined as:

$$E = \frac{abs(logP \sim logD)}{\alpha1\ +\ (\alpha2 + \alpha3) \cdot (\frac{\beta}{abs(logP \sim logD)})) + (1 - exp(-\frac{abs(logP \sim logD)}{\beta})) - (\alpha3 * exp(-\frac{abs(logP \sim logD)}{\beta}))}$$

The NSS model was calibrated using the zero rate. Because the result was observed at the maximum hydrophobicity impact on the ligand, the maturity parameter in the NSS model was replaced by the hydrophobicity parameter. It was important to note that the extent of hydrophobicity was planned at a pH equal to 7.0. Because of the hydrophobicity of the binding pocket, the NSS model equation derivative at a tenor point represents a featured value for ligand-protein interaction. Binding site residues induce hydrophobic involvement within the binding pocket, where the ligand has accumulated binding opportunities. However, it is impossible to quantify the extent to which hydrophobicity influences ligand attraction during molecular interaction. To address this issue, the hydrophobicity value was assumed based on the ligand itself. It was also assumed that when ligand-protein interactions occur as a result of the hydrophobicity of the binding site, the maximum attraction attained on the ligand must be a function of the hydrophobicity calculated for the ligand. It was also assumed that the distance between the binding site and the ligand could represent the extent of molecular interaction. The distance between the centroids of the binding site and the ligand was used to present this parameter. For the parameters governing the relationship between hydrophobicity and the distance between the centroids, the NSS model derivative for zero rates was simulated. Because it was assumed that the calculated hydrophobicity value for ligand will represent the maximum attraction between ligand and protein, the maturity parameter was replaced by hydrophobicity. The NSS model distribution was found to be followed by the simulated efficacy of ligands. A real ligand-receptor interaction was then evaluated to determine the dependability of the customised model. In this case, the receptor was a binding pocket on a virus's glycoprotein spikes, and the ligand was a receptor determinant present on the host's cell surface. This study used one naturally occurring receptor determinant, along with analogues derived from the pharmacophore of the virus's binding pocket at the glycoprotein spike. It was assumed that the naturally occurring receptor determinant would outperform the majority of the analogues, and if any analogue outperforms the naturally occurring receptor determinant, then the receptor determinant may be a new possibility to prove competition with the natural receptor determinant.

Validation and Case Study

Binding site domain, pharmacophore, and identified receptor determinant analogues were taken into account from DOI: 10.26434/chemrxiv.12241634.v1; where a study was conducted to identify possible receptor determinant analogues for all 9-O-Ac-Sialoglycan-Recognizing Coronaviruses. The binding pocket, in this case, had two domains, P1 and P2. The initial protein and ligand dataset were adapted from DOI: 10.26434/chemrxiv.12241634.v1. Both binding pockets were simulated, and different kinetics model parameter values were discovered (Table 1). The rate of viral infectivity was shown to be a direct result of Ligand's ability to chase Viral Spike. Naturally, known receptor determinants were found to be far more effective than the vast majority of analogues identified *via* the same pharmacophore. This case study validated the dependability of customised kinetic models.

Table 1. Model parameters have been optimised for two domains, P1 and P2.

Parameter	Domain P1
α 1	-465.707091
α 2	474.1327822

(Table 1) cont.....

Parameter	Domain P1
α 3	540.5571268
β	16.38474885

Parameter	Domain P2
α 1	-478.0579251
α 2	484.9847989
α 3	518.7311.35
β	22.36179227

Prioritization of Receptor Determinant Analogues: Anti-corona virus receptor determinant analogues discovered in DOI: 10.26434/chemrxiv.12241634.v1 were evaluated using system models of two binding site domains. A comparison of phase plots revealed that ligands were causing un-stability in virus spikes (Figs. **2 - 7**). Because two different domains were active, no stable null point was achieved. Analogue C3 was found to be equivalent to receptor determinants in terms of performance. As a result, C3 has antiviral activity.

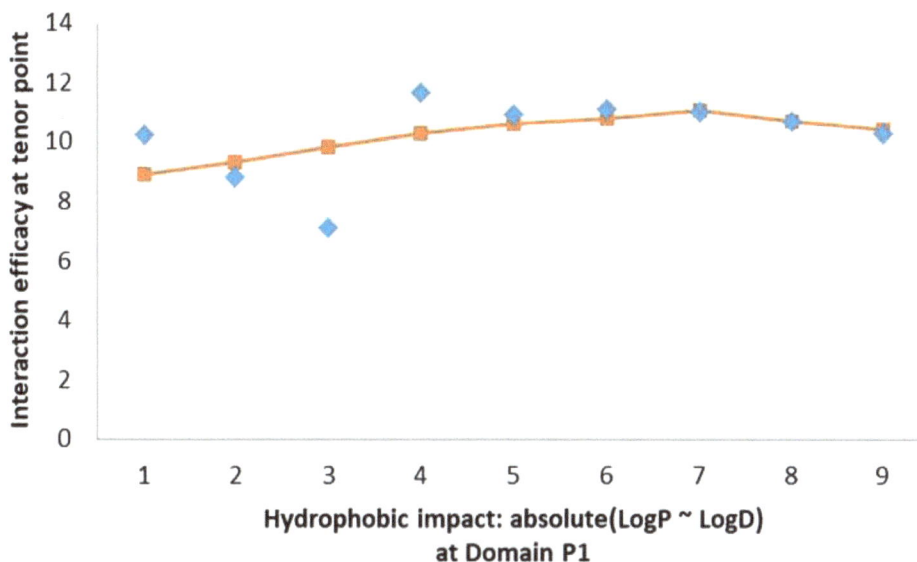

Fig. (3A). The rate of viral infectivity has been shown to be a direct result of ligand's ability to chase viral spike at domain P1.

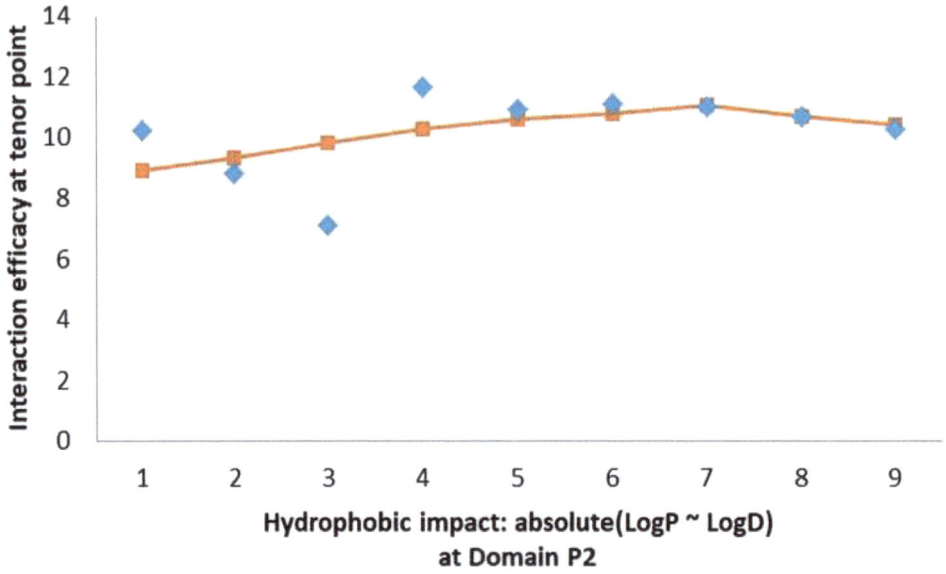

Fig. (3B). The rate of viral infectivity can be shown to be a direct result of ligand's ability to chase viral spike at domain P2.

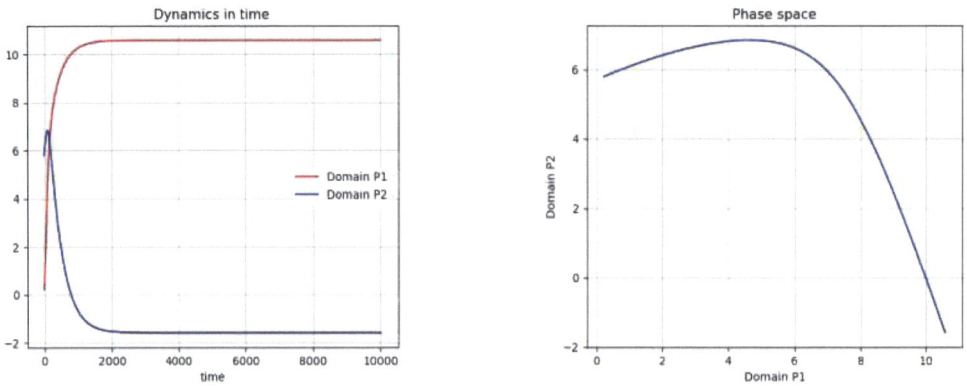

Fig. (4). A broad view of a system with two domains, P1 and P2, interacting with receptor determinants.

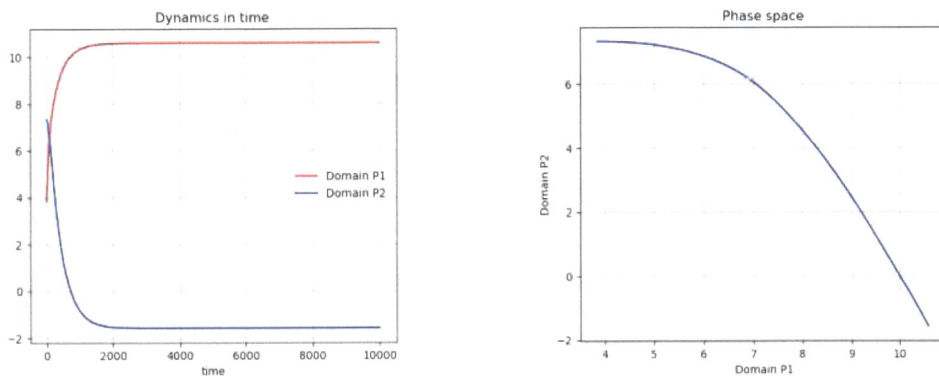

Fig. (5). Co-Crystallized Ligand of 6NZK.

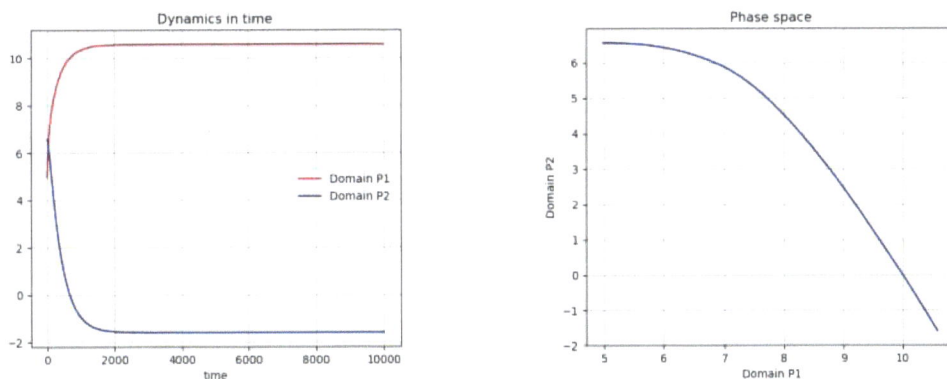

Fig. (6). C3's performance is comparable to that of a receptor determinant.

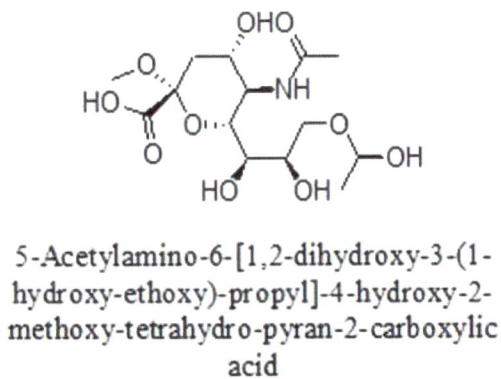

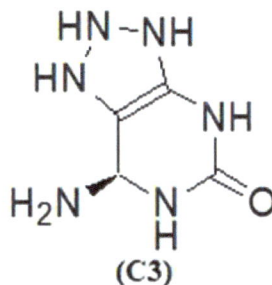

5-Acetylamino-6-[1,2-dihydroxy-3-(1-hydroxy-ethoxy)-propyl]-4-hydroxy-2-methoxy-tetrahydro-pyran-2-carboxylic acid

(C3)

Fig. (7). C3 as a prioritised analogue of a natural receptor determinant.

Repurposing through Electronic Health Records

Pathological records (numerical) can be another basis for drug repurposing. Since the main attention is on the observations of the impact of drugs on various physiological states. That means if we observe a significant difference in two observations of a physiological parameter due to the use of a specific prescription; it will be an indication of drug repositioning possibilities. Such types of observations are performed through the baseline regularization model using electronic health records (EHRs) [17]. In EHRs, drug prescriptions are noted down along with pathological measurements (*e.g.*, blood sugar, *etc.*) of patients throughout the time. Under this method, fluctuations in pathological measurements are observed; and statistical analysis is performed with the use of a particular drug. This process helps in the identification of potential repurposing opportunities [18].

RECENT ADVANCEMENTS IN AI ALGORITHMS FOR DRUG REPURPOSING

Deep learning allows researchers to find multi-modal biomarkers to develop more effective and personalized treatments, early diagnosis tools, as well as useful information for drug discovery and repurposing in neurodegenerative pathologies. It significantly accelerates the drug discovery process and contributes to global efforts to stop the spread of infectious diseases. It can also be used to find less toxic drug through repurposed drugs [19].

Machine learning is successful when well-defined featured data is available for model development. In the context of data analysis for drug-repurposing, the organization of the hierarchy of the data as well as its transformation, is at the core. This architecture of a multi-level data structure generates patterns during model training, which is captured through a subfield of machine learning methods known as deep learning. Perceptron performs the basic data transformation process, which is the unit component of an artificial neural network [20]. It is to notify you that ANN is the most diversely implemented method in deep learning. Perceptrons are known as unit-artificial neurons. A bunch of perceptrons creates an interconnected network, which receives raw inputs and transforms them through multi-layered as well as interconnected layers named 'hidden' & 'output' layers. This architecture is called a feed-forward neural network. The forwarded information from the output layer is sent back for evaluation and correction of memory; this process is called backpropagation. Both the process of feed-forward and backpropagation are repeated multiple times to stabilize the memory weights at the minimum loss of the information. It is to notify that the input layer of neurons receives a vector as input. Three main artificial intelligence methods are used for drug repurposing: Artificial Neural network, Convolutional Neural Network, and Recurrent Neural Network [21]. For example, if you want to train a model for the classification of drugs based on pharmaceutical performance, then the RNA expression vector of multiple genes can be considered as input. Similarly, if you want to predict the possible performance of the drugs based on structures, then molecular descriptors along with target information should be considered as input.

There are some cases where weighted memory size becomes very large, in those cases, small matrices are used as filters for input data. These matrices are implemented for windowed matrix multiplication to transform into lightweight data. An example of such a case is image processing through convolutional neural networks (CNN). Similarly, molecular interaction between ligand and protein is also processed through CNN models. Beyond these, sequences are also used for drug repurposing. Sequence data is trained with recurrent neural networks (RNNs). RNN is used for capturing patterns hidden in data series. An important feature of RNN (beyond the above methods) is the retention of record memory, which makes RNN valuable for drug-target interaction as well as other processes where inputs come in the form of line entry sequences. Besides individual attempts, hybrids of feed-forward & RNN; and hybrids of CNN & RNN were known to be used for the development of anti-SARS-CoV-2 drugs [22].

Graph Representation Learning

The graph-based method is used for establishing relationships among the data nodes with a very high number along with low dimensional feature vectors. This method predicts possible links among the components. Network medicine is one of the most suited examples in the area of medical knowledge analysis. For drug repurposing (*e.g.*, for COVID-19), the medical knowledge entities, *i.e.*, feature components, are used to establish relationships among a set of drugs and pharmaceutical aspects. Similarity and dissimilarity are calculated based on feature components. Scalability is a challenge in graph-based methods. The real-world medical data size is quite large, several million. Therefore, enhancements are being made for handling such a large size of data. For regular purposes, TensorFlow and PyTorch are used, while for large data sizes, GraphVite is used. These developments encourage the enthusiasm for developing enhanced graph learning methods. As for relating drug-vs-disease, knowledge graphs have been developed based on literature data regarding drugs, disease, genes, and protein, *etc*. In another study graph, the neural network has been utilized for the identification of repurposed drugs against SARS-CoV-2.

REPURPOSED-DRUG THERAPIES UNDER INVESTIGATION AGAINST COVID-19

Although examples as well as detailed discussion, are available for repurposed drugs against COVID-1-9. Here, we will revisit a few of them for repurposing aspects in terms of existing drugs, launched due to the computational efficiency of implementing advanced methods.

Therapy Targeting Virus

Considering the knowledge-based discovery, inhibition of viral RNA polymerase for the development of antiviral drugs was revisited by FDA. A drug, already known against the Ebola virus, was proposed against COVID-19 [23]. It was 'Remdesivir'. It significantly shortened the median recovery time of patients. A machine learning approach was utilized to discover 'Mefuparib' to block replication of SARS-CoV-2 at the early infection stage [24]. It was found mechanistically similar to Rendesivir for the post-entry stage. Network medicine analysis as well as biophysics-based theoretical studies, suggested antiviral activity of 'Toremifene' as potent against COVID-19, by blocking ACE2 and the spike protein of the virus; while it is already a well-known anti-cancer molecule.

The new therapeutic opportunities were observed based on corticosteroids, RNA polymerase, interferons, protease, and some others. Novel drug candidates have been suggested on the basis of the SARS-CoV-2-host protein interaction network, spike surface glycoprotein and RNA polymerase. SARS-CoV-2 RNA-dependent RNA polymerase (RdRp) is almost preserved across different viral species and can be a potential target for the development of antiviral drugs, including nucleoside analogs [25]. Another important benefit is that viral RNA-polymerase has no counterpart in human cells, which makes it an excellent target. Although different types of antiviral targets are applicable for SARS-CoV-2 drug screenings, the promising targets were considered as 3C-like main protease (3Cl protease) and RNA polymerase. Considering these aspects, genomic insights into understanding the structure-function relationships of drug targets, including spike, main protease, and RNA-dependent RNA polymerase of SARS-CoV-2, have been discussed intensively. The drugs such as Favipiravir and Lopinavir/Ritonavir under the antiviral category, the angiotensin-converting enzyme 2 (the renin-angiotensin system inhibitors), Remdesivir (RNA polymerase inhibitor) from the antiviral category, cepharanthine from the anti-inflammatory category, *etc.*, are still under consideration [26]. These drugs target three major processes: (1) the early stages of virus-cell interaction, (2) viral proteases, and (3) the viral RNA-dependent RNA polymerase. RNA polymerase and spike glycoprotein were also tested *in vitro* and/or in clinical trials as well as on promising compounds proven to be active against coronaviruses by an *in-silico* drug repurposing approach. However, there are therapeutic drugs with the potential to inhibit endocytic pathways, suppress ribonucleic acid (RNA) polymerase activities, and reduce the replication of SARS-CoV-2.

Therapy Targeting Host

Although large-scale evaluation is still on wait, therapeutic attempts have also been made by targeting the host. It is well known that COVID-19-infected patients bear severe systemic inflammation and a cytokine storm. By implementing network medicine-based big data analysis, a few known drugs (*e.g.*, Baricitinib, Dexamethasone, Melatonin, *etc.*) were tried for anti-inflammatory and immune response against COVID-19. Few positive results were found, but still, large-scale population data is not available [27].

Breaking and reinvestigating mechanisms of action could provide new insights for the identification of new leads. Recent strategies in antiviral research are based on the identification of molecules targeting host functions required for the infection of multiple viruses. Repurposed antivirals have been categorised into two major groups: (i) direct-acting repurposed antivirals (DARA) and (ii) host-targeting repurposed antivirals (HTRA). But in general, antiviral targets can be considered as targeting the host or the host's immune cells [28].

Compounds that exert their antiviral activities mainly through host factors and immunomodulation, such as host targeting agents (HTAs), programmed cell death protein 1 (PD-1)/programmed death-ligand 1 (PD-L1) inhibitors, and Toll-like receptor (TLR) agonists, were also considered [29]. These novel antiviral molecules, in combination with conventional antiviral agents targeting the virus, will ideally enter the clinics and reinforce the therapeutic arsenal to combat influenza virus infections.

In particular, drug repurposing has been adopted as a validated method for saving time and cost relative to the traditional development of drugs. Algorithms like CoVex are involved in a therapeutic chase against COVID-19. Beyond these, alternative approaches are also being utilised for the inhibition of activity. In a study, host-directed TB therapies targeting pro- or anti-inflammatory processes have been evaluated in pre-clinical models. Host-targeting cross-protective efficacy of anticoagulants against SARS-CoV-2 was also used. In this way, strategies targeting both virus and host factors have been pursued to identify broad-spectrum anti-flavivirus agents [30].

Therapy through Drug Combinations

Drug repurposing, involving the identification of single or combinations of existing drugs based on human genetics data and network biology approaches, represents a next-generation approach that has the potential to increase the speed of drug discovery at a lower cost [31]. It screens synergistic drug combinations for infectious diseases. It can encourage novel therapeutics against remerging viruses. Repurposed and combination therapies are also an eye target for rapid implementation [32].

Beyond the little to no benefit of suggested monotherapies of Remedesivir, Mefuparib, Toremifene, Baricitinib, Dexamethasone, Melatonin, Baricitinib, *etc.*; drug combinations were also tried. Drug combinations against COVID-19 were identified through interactome network-based methods. A few identified combinations were as: (i) Remdesivir with Baricitinib, (ii) Sirolimus with Dactinomycin, (iii) Mercaptopurine with Melatonin, (iv) Toremifene with Emodin, (v) Melatonin and Toremifene and, (vi) Baricitinib + Remdesivir [22].

CHALLENGES IN RE-INSIGHT FOR DRUG REPURPOSING

Along with the benefits of drug-repurposing, there are many turning point challenges also. These challenges may be at the experimental level; that means during the discovery of repurposed drugs, there are factors related to environmental constraints which become absent during any type of laboratory experiments in the laboratory. Although we are trying to speak out about the power of repurposed-drug from the existing ones, we do not involve the contribution of those factors that link the drugs with the environment. In this way, we are missing the connectivity between the drug and its relative impact to and fro with the environmental constraints. In this way, we find that the discovered drug may be considered a repurposed drug. But in many aspects, we will miss out on the factors from the clinical-side also. That means, when we will implement the drug, we will definitely not be able to avail of the clinical benefits [33].

Beyond the above-discussed missing points, other questions also put repurposed drugs out of the circle, when we think about more biologically. The reason behind it is that we do not know the possible behaviour of repurposed drugs during molecular interactions as well as in all related experiments [34].

As the scientific attitude of any research is accepted on the criteria of statistical significance, but in the case of repurposed drugs, statistics of significance are not managed. Because we didn't follow the evidence related to drug *versus* patient or there is very little data related to patients and that drug for specific purposes [35].

Another critical drawback comes into existence when we do not receive reproducible results during clinical trials. The reason behind it is the same, as we discussed above, that we are missing the various aspects related to drugs and their significant use under constraints. These aspects are related to the local biological system at a specific person where we try to implement a repurposed drug, but when we think about the implementation of such drugs at the population level, another constraint comes into existence; that is the diversity in the genetic behavior in the population. Variation of genetic background in the population makes the repurposed drug motivating the researchers to understand the distribution of population in relation to the reuse of the discovered drugs, so it becomes necessary to rethink about use of drugs in the population [36].

Diversity in the population also pushes the observers to make wrong pathological decisions. Since the data generated during the pathological testing remain very small, therefore the decision-making data distribution does not exist, which makes the observer move in the wrong direction [37].

As we know, any disease grows from a normal state to an advanced state; that indicates the possibility of multiple stages during the development of the disease. The use of drugs varies from one stage to another stage. Since the repurposed drug is not identified or linked with the stage of disease, therefore this situation becomes another constraint for the use of repurposed drugs.

Beyond the above-discussed point of challenges, one more challenge came into existence when we observed the pharmacological aspects (*i.e.*, Pharmacodynamics and pharmacokinetics) related to drugs and the human body.

So, although we are claiming about the discovery of the purpose drugs for various diseases as well as covid-19, with the help of artificial intelligence, in many aspects, we are not able to provide the required information to our developing artificial intelligence system for identifying real implementable repurposed drugs.

The reason behind the development of an incomplete AI model for drug repurposing is the unavailability of data representing the complexity of hierarchically regulated biological systems. These AI algorithms are capable of capturing the patterns from multi-level interactions and developing suitable systems for handling complex systems. In this development, there is an additional constraint in the form of normalizing data from different sources for different populations. That means the arrangement of biological data and formation from molecular to population level in a synchronized manner is today's biggest problem for the development of artificial intelligence-based systems for drug repurposing. The requirement of availability of such data-driven information is not being completed because of the socio-ethical aspects also [38].

Challenges in Data Sharing and Security

This socio-ethical aspect is directly linked with ethical issues related to the collection of patient-specific pathological evidence. Legally, expressing the identity of the patient is not valid. Another aspect is that each patient cannot be used as a volunteer for the collection of every aspect of biological data related to drug development. That means, we directly cannot perform molecular to population-level experiments with every patient at different geographical locations. Then what may be the solution for fulfilling the benefits of the discovery of repurposed drugs? There may be one suggestive solution in the form of federated learning: that means if every individual becomes aware of providing the individual status of their health, disease, and the treatment journey evidence through the digital devices through individual mobile phones are local servers extra. In this way, the collection of the data will be in a structured format, as well as the information of the individual persons will be in encrypted form. Only the well-trained models will be opened for use in scientific development. In this way, this data security and individual privacy will be maintained, and it will also support the fast development of repurposed drugs [39].

PERSONALISED AND AI-GUIDED REPURPOSING

The term 'personalized', in the area of disease therapeutics, is directly linked with the profile of the gene set of an individual. Here, the word profile is used in terms of an individual's genetic behavior of genes. The benefits of such profiles were utilized in the preciseness of some disease therapeutics. As in the case of cancer, the effect of drugs was observed with the genetic, epigenetic, and environmental factors. Since, in the case of COVID-19 infection, high variability was observed among populations, the implementation of personalized thinking for drug repurposing is assumed to have an impact. Therefore, observation of human genetics of the population might be used for understanding the clinical characteristics as well as the response of the drug. In a population experiment with >80,000 genomes, it was observed that the SARS-CoV-2 infected population without expression of TMPRSS2 benefited from hydroxychloroquine or chloroquine. This experiment was successful in case of viral infection in the kidney, but not in nasal or bronchial cells and lung. The point of attention is that these studies established the importance of pharmacogenomics in the enhancement of clinical basis for personalised treatment, although data for COVID-19 therapy are limited to define the success stories. AI techniques can be used to determine the genetic basis of SARS-CoV-2 pathogenesis, followed by repurposed personalised treatment of COVID-19. AI integrates multi-strata experimental data, followed by feature extraction, to picturise output for personalized drug repurposing [40].

CONCLUSION

Future AI-informed drug repurposing can be imagined as the requirement-dependent discovery of a drug. AI will show its potential to pick out existing drugs for different purposes, as new health issues will come into existence, saying in brief that uncertainty of time for identification of drugs will be minimized. Because of defined methods, newly repurposed drugs will be processed and crossed rapidly at various levels of clinical trials. This process will also generate a large amount of data in the area of *in-vitro*, *in-vivo* experiments, and reported scientific literature. The deposited huge data will make AI more capable of making efficient decisions. These collected data will also be useful to experts from different areas. With these views, AI is being considered a background force for enhancing the speed of drug repurposing, including COVID-19. Along with these possible opportunities, various challenges will remain in existence during the whole process of discovery of AI-guided selective therapeutics as; as quality & diversity of data, and insufficient & insecure sharing of data and models. Under light of existing evidence, the expectation arises for the development of accurate AI models for drug repurposing to generate outcomes.

CONSENT FOR PUBLICATION

Not applicable.

CONFLICT OF INTEREST

The authors declare no conflict of interest, financial or otherwise.

ACKNOWLEDGEMENTS

Authors are thankful to the Director, CSIR-Central Institute of Medicinal & Aromatic Plants (CIMAP), Lucknow, India for infrastructure & research facilities support. Author OP is thankful to the Indian Council of Medical Research (ICMR), New Delhi, India for financial support through RA fellowship (Award letter no. BMI/11(12)/2020, dated: 04/02/2021) The CSIR-CIMAP Communication Number is CIMAP/PUB/2022/120.

REFERENCES

[1]   Carroll J. One drug, many uses. Biotechnol Healthc 2005; 2(5): 56-61.
[PMID: 23424312]

[2]   Sahoo BM, Ravi Kumar BVV, Sruti J, Mahapatra MK, Banik BK, Borah P. Drug Repurposing Strategy (DRS): Emerging Approach to Identify Potential Therapeutics for Treatment of Novel Coronavirus Infection. Front Mol Biosci 2021; 8: 628144.
[http://dx.doi.org/10.3389/fmolb.2021.628144] [PMID: 33718434]

[3]   Csermely P, Korcsmáros T, Kiss HJM, London G, Nussinov R. Structure and dynamics of molecular

networks: A novel paradigm of drug discovery. Pharmacol Ther 2013; 138(3): 333-408.
[http://dx.doi.org/10.1016/j.pharmthera.2013.01.016] [PMID: 23384594]

[4]   Dudley JT, Deshpande T, Butte AJ. Exploiting drug-disease relationships for computational drug repositioning. Brief Bioinform 2011; 12(4): 303-11.
[http://dx.doi.org/10.1093/bib/bbr013] [PMID: 21690101]

[5]   Schadt EE, Linderman MD, Sorenson J, Lee L, Nolan GP. Computational solutions to large-scale data management and analysis. Nat Rev Genet 2010; 11(9): 647-57.
[http://dx.doi.org/10.1038/nrg2857] [PMID: 20717155]

[6]   Sohraby F, Bagheri M, Aryapour H. Performing an *in silico* repurposing of existing drugs by combining virtual screening and molecular dynamics simulation. Methods Mol Biol 2019; 1903: 23-43.
[http://dx.doi.org/10.1007/978-1-4939-8955-3_2] [PMID: 30547434]

[7]   Udrescu M, Udrescu L. A Drug Repurposing Method Based on Drug-Drug Interaction Networks and Using Energy Model Layouts. Methods Mol Biol 2019; 1903: 185-201.
[http://dx.doi.org/10.1007/978-1-4939-8955-3_11] [PMID: 30547443]

[8]   Rodriguez S, Hug C, Todorov P, *et al.* Machine learning identifies candidates for drug repurposing in Alzheimer's disease. Nat Commun 2021; 12(1): 1033.
[http://dx.doi.org/10.1038/s41467-021-21330-0] [PMID: 33589615]

[9]   Deb S, Reeves AA. Simulation of Remdesivir Pharmacokinetics and Its Drug Interactions. J Pharm Pharm Sci 2021; 24: 277-91.
[http://dx.doi.org/10.18433/jpps32011] [PMID: 34107241]

[10]   Jain S, Potschka H, Chandra PP, Tripathi M, Vohora D. Management of COVID-19 in patients with seizures: Mechanisms of action of potential COVID-19 drug treatments and consideration for potential drug-drug interactions with anti-seizure medications. Epilepsy Res 2021; 174: 106675.
[http://dx.doi.org/10.1016/j.eplepsyres.2021.106675] [PMID: 34044300]

[11]   Nascimento ACA, Prudêncio RBC, Costa IG. A Drug-Target Network-Based Supervised Machine Learning Repurposing Method Allowing the Use of Multiple Heterogeneous Information Sources. Methods Mol Biol 2019; 1903: 281-9.
[http://dx.doi.org/10.1007/978-1-4939-8955-3_17] [PMID: 30547449]

[12]   Vogrinc D, Kunej T. Drug repositioning: computational approaches and research examples classified according to the evidence level. Discoveries (Craiova) 2017; 5(2): e75.
[http://dx.doi.org/10.15190/d.2017.5] [PMID: 32309593]

[13]   Zheng S, Ma H, Wang J, Li J. A Computational Bipartite Graph-Based Drug Repurposing Method. Methods Mol Biol 2019; 1903: 115-27.
[http://dx.doi.org/10.1007/978-1-4939-8955-3_7] [PMID: 30547439]

[14]   Ginex T, Garaigorta U, Ramírez D, *et al.* Host-Directed FDA-Approved Drugs with Antiviral Activity against SARS-CoV-2 Identified by Hierarchical In Silico/*In Vitro* Screening Methods. Pharmaceuticals (Basel) 2021; 14(4): 332.
[http://dx.doi.org/10.3390/ph14040332] [PMID: 33917313]

[15]   Maurya PP. Receptor Determinant Analogues for All 9-O-Ac-Sialoglycan-Recognizing Corona Viruses. ChemRxiv Cambridge Open Engage 2020.
[http://dx.doi.org/10.26434/chemrxiv.12241634.v1]

[16]   Prakash O. Hydrophobicity as a Parameter to Quantify Relative Efficacy of Receptor Determinants During Host Virus Interaction. ChemRxiv Cambridge Open Engage 2020.
[http://dx.doi.org/10.26434/chemrxiv.12424376.v1]

[17]   Kuang Z, Bao Y, Thomson J, *et al.* A Machine-Learning-Based Drug Repurposing Approach Using Baseline Regularization. Methods Mol Biol 2019; 1903: 255-67.
[http://dx.doi.org/10.1007/978-1-4939-8955-3_15] [PMID: 30547447]

[18]   Ahmed Z, Mohamed K, Zeeshan S, Dong X. Artificial intelligence with multi-functional machine learning platform development for better healthcare and precision medicine. Database (Oxford) 2020; 2020: baaa010.
[http://dx.doi.org/10.1093/database/baaa010] [PMID: 32185396]

[19]   Vamathevan J, Clark D, Czodrowski P, *et al.* Applications of machine learning in drug discovery and development. Nat Rev Drug Discov 2019; 18(6): 463-77.
[http://dx.doi.org/10.1038/s41573-019-0024-5] [PMID: 30976107]

[20]   Tanoli Z, Vähä-Koskela M, Aittokallio T. Artificial intelligence, machine learning, and drug repurposing in cancer. Expert Opin Drug Discov 2021; 16(9): 977-89.
[http://dx.doi.org/10.1080/17460441.2021.1883585] [PMID: 33543671]

[21]   Tian Q, Ding M, Yang H, *et al.* Predicting drug-target affinity based on recurrent neural networks and graph convolutional neural networks. Comb Chem High Throughput Screen 2021. Epub ahead of print
[http://dx.doi.org/10.2174/1386207324666210215101825] [PMID: 33588722]

[22]   Zhou Y, Wang F, Tang J, Nussinov R, Cheng F. Artificial intelligence in COVID-19 drug repurposing. Lancet Digit Health 2020; 2(12): e667-76.
[http://dx.doi.org/10.1016/S2589-7500(20)30192-8] [PMID: 32984792]

[23]   Dotolo S, Marabotti A, Facchiano A, Tagliaferri R. A review on drug repurposing applicable to COVID-19. Brief Bioinform 2021; 22(2): 726-41.
[http://dx.doi.org/10.1093/bib/bbaa288] [PMID: 33147623]

[24]   Ge Y, Tian T, Huang S, *et al.* An integrative drug repositioning framework discovered a potential therapeutic agent targeting COVID-19. Signal Transduct Target Ther 2021; 6(1): 165.
[http://dx.doi.org/10.1038/s41392-021-00568-6] [PMID: 33895786]

[25]   Kifle ZD, Ayele AG, Enyew EF. Drug Repurposing Approach, Potential Drugs, and Novel Drug Targets for COVID-19 Treatment. J Environ Public Health 2021; 2021: 1-11.
[http://dx.doi.org/10.1155/2021/6631721] [PMID: 33953756]

[26]   Poduri R, Joshi G, Jagadeesh G. Drugs targeting various stages of the SARS-CoV-2 life cycle: Exploring promising drugs for the treatment of Covid-19. Cell Signal 2020; 74: 109721.
[http://dx.doi.org/10.1016/j.cellsig.2020.109721] [PMID: 32711111]

[27]   Zhu Y, Li J, Pang Z. Recent insights for the emerging COVID-19: Drug discovery, therapeutic options and vaccine development. Asian Journal of Pharmaceutical Sciences 2021; 16(1): 4-23.
[http://dx.doi.org/10.1016/j.ajps.2020.06.001] [PMID: 32837565]

[28]   Ullah H, Hou W, Dakshanamurthy S, Tang Q. Host targeted antiviral (HTA): functional inhibitor compounds of scaffold protein RACK1 inhibit herpes simplex virus proliferation. Oncotarget 2019; 10(35): 3209-26.
[http://dx.doi.org/10.18632/oncotarget.26907] [PMID: 31143369]

[29]   Zhang N, Tu J, Wang X, Chu Q. Programmed cell death-1/programmed cell death ligand-1 checkpoint inhibitors: differences in mechanism of action. Immunotherapy 2019; 11(5): 429-41.
[http://dx.doi.org/10.2217/imt-2018-0110] [PMID: 30698054]

[30]   Fiscon G, Conte F, Farina L, Paci P. SAveRUNNER: A network-based algorithm for drug repurposing and its application to COVID-19. PLOS Comput Biol 2021; 17(2): e1008686.
[http://dx.doi.org/10.1371/journal.pcbi.1008686] [PMID: 33544720]

[31]   Zheng W, Sun W, Simeonov A. Drug repurposing screens and synergistic drug-combinations for infectious diseases. Br J Pharmacol 2018; 175(2): 181-91.
[http://dx.doi.org/10.1111/bph.13895] [PMID: 28685814]

[32]   Xu T, Zheng W, Huang R. High-throughput screening assays for SARS-CoV-2 drug development: Current status and future directions. Drug Discov Today 2021; 26(10): 2439-44.
[http://dx.doi.org/10.1016/j.drudis.2021.05.012] [PMID: 34048893]

[33]   Parvathaneni V, Gupta V. Utilizing drug repurposing against COVID-19 – Efficacy, limitations, and challenges. Life Sci 2020; 259: 118275.
[http://dx.doi.org/10.1016/j.lfs.2020.118275] [PMID: 32818545]

[34]   Cha Y, Erez T, Reynolds IJ, *et al.* Drug repurposing from the perspective of pharmaceutical companies. Br J Pharmacol 2018; 175(2): 168-80.
[http://dx.doi.org/10.1111/bph.13798] [PMID: 28369768]

[35]   McLellan AT. Substance Misuse and Substance use Disorders: Why do they Matter in Healthcare? Trans Am Clin Climatol Assoc 2017; 128: 112-30.
[PMID: 28790493]

[36]   Fogel DB. Factors associated with clinical trials that fail and opportunities for improving the likelihood of success: A review. Contemp Clin Trials Commun 2018; 11: 156-64.
[http://dx.doi.org/10.1016/j.conctc.2018.08.001] [PMID: 30112460]

[37]   Mooney SWJ, Alam NM, Prusky GT. Tracking-Based Interactive Assessment of Saccades, Pursuits, Visual Field, and Contrast Sensitivity in Children With Brain Injury. Front Hum Neurosci 2021; 15: 737409.
[http://dx.doi.org/10.3389/fnhum.2021.737409] [PMID: 34776907]

[38]   Bohr A, Memarzadeh K. The rise of artificial intelligence in healthcare applications 2020; 25-60.
[http://dx.doi.org/10.1016/B978-0-12-818438-7.00002-2]

[39]   Pushpakom S, Iorio F, Eyers PA, *et al.* Drug repurposing: progress, challenges and recommendations. Nat Rev Drug Discov 2019; 18(1): 41-58.
[http://dx.doi.org/10.1038/nrd.2018.168] [PMID: 30310233]

[40]   Levin JM, Oprea TI, Davidovich S, *et al.* Artificial intelligence, drug repurposing and peer review. Nat Biotechnol 2020; 38(10): 1127-31.
[http://dx.doi.org/10.1038/s41587-020-0686-x] [PMID: 32929264]

SUBJECT INDEX

www.ingramcontent.com/pod-product-compliance
Lightning Source LLC
Chambersburg PA
CBHW041659210326
41598CB00007B/465